Be a Survivor™

Your Guide to Breast Cancer Treatment

Third Edition
Fully Revised

Be a Survivor™
Your Guide to Breast Cancer Treatment — 3rd ed.

Vladimir Lange, M.D.

ISBN 0-9663610-8-3

Second printing, April, 2006

A CIP record for this book is available from the Library of Congress.

Printed in the United States of America

Be a Survivor™

Your Guide to Breast Cancer Treatment

Third Edition
Fully Revised

VLADIMIR LANGE, M.D.

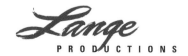

PRODUCTIONS

LOS ANGELES

To Mandy,
Chad, and Christy

Credits

Cover Art:
Lily Kovacevik

Graphic Artists:
Tim Doherty
Scott Gray
Nigel Lizaranzu
Brooks Rawlins

Contributing Writer:
Christina Lange

Photography:
Steven Bradford
Chad Lange

Reviewers:
William H. Goodson III, MD
Anne Mercer Larson
Cathy Masamitsu
Candace Moorman, MPH
Carol Reed

Table of Contents

CONSULTANTS FOR *BE A SURVIVOR*

**This book was developed with the invaluable assistance
of the following leading experts:**

Terri Ades, M.S., R.N.
Leslie Botnick, M.D.
R. James Brenner, M.D., J.D.
Kristin Brill, M.D.
Aman Buzdar, M.D.
Cathy Coleman, R.N., O.C.N.
Helen Crothers, M.S.W.
Bradford W. Edgerton, M.D.
Barbara Fowble, M.D.
William H. Goodson, III, M.D.
William H. Hindle, M.D.
Soram Singh Khalsa, M.D.
Lydia Komarnicky, M.D.
Joshua Levine, M.D.
Silvana Martino, D.O.
Stephen Mathes, M.D.
Beatrice Mautner, R.N.
Shirley McKenzie, R.N., P.H.N.
Candace Moorman, M.P.H.
Betsy Mullen
Anne Rosenberg, M.D.
Christy A. Russell, M.D.
Karen Schmitt, R.N.
Stuart J. Schnitt, M.D.
Barbara L. Smith, M.D., Ph.D.
David Spiegel, M.D.
Lisa Summerlot, R.N., O.C.N.
Marilou Terpenning, M.D.
Victor Vogel, M.D.
Deane Wolcott, M.D.

Acknowledgments

This book is based on more than a decade of professional experience creating educational programs about breast cancer, and on my personal experience dealing with breast cancer as the husband of a survivor.

A list of the names of all those who helped me, encouraged me, and taught me during these years would be longer than the book itself. I thank all of them for their time and kind support.

Several of them deserve special gratitude.

My most sincere thanks go to my valued consultants, recognized experts in their fields, who contributed their time and knowledge to make this book informative, accurate, and up-to-date. It is particularly gratifying that two of them, William Goodson and David Spiegel, are my friends and classmates from Harvard Medical School days. Bill reviewed the manuscript from cover to cover, with surgical precision, spotting areas that needed enhancement.

Three of the consultants, Lisa Summerlot, Karen Schmitt, and Candace Moorman, contributed their extensive experience in dealing with breast cancer patients. They helped me not only with the facts, but also with my writing style.

Lisa helped write the scripts and overcome the production stumbling blocks for many of the video programs on which the CD-ROM and the book are based.

Karen reviewed the entire CD-ROM from introduction to credits, mercilessly pointing out where my style did not measure up.

And Candace challenged me by saying that the world did not need another breast cancer book, then rewarded me by admitting that she wished she had this book when she was diagnosed with breast cancer herself.

Thank you! Each of you made the book better.

I also want to thank the survivors and their families, who gave freely of their time and candidly shared their stories. Two survivors deserve extra special thanks.

Betsy Mullen, diagnosed at age 33, contributed her experience, not only as a survivor, but also as the founder and president of WIN, the Women's Information Network Against Breast Cancer. Cathy Masamitsu, diagnosed at age 32, helped bring the *Be A Survivor* program to the attention of her viewers on the *Home & Family Show.*

Thanks to my efficient and talented team for working so diligently during production of all the programs on which this book is based. Special thanks to Jim Robie of Los Angeles for generously contributing his talent in creating the design and layout for the book.

My deep gratitude to Carol Reed who contributed her extensive experience and boundless energy to make the launch of this third edition a success.

My love and gratitude to our children, Chad and Christy, for always being there for me, for their Mom, and for each other. And most of all, my love and admiration to Mandy, who has survived her battle with breast cancer and remains in my life as a shining beacon, a powerful inspiration, and a valued critic.

Introduction
to the Third Edition

It has been gratifying to see *Be a Survivor* grow from a modest addition to a long list of excellent books on breast cancer, to a unique patient education system that includes videos, DVD's, CD-ROM's, and much-needed Spanish versions of the program. These *Be a Survivor* products have won many awards for excellence, and have been widely distributed throughout the country and around the world.

Even more gratifying is the feedback from readers. "Best ever...," "My constant companion...," "Great explanation of a very complex subject." These comments make me feel that as a physician, as a writer, and as the husband of a breast cancer survivor, I have helped relieve the pain and confusion inflicted by this disease.

Five years after the publication of the first edition, the vast majority of the women featured in the book are alive and well. And so is my wife, 16 years after her diagnosis, now as strong and healthy as ever.

It is regrettable that this third edition was not rendered unnecessary by some newly-discovered cure for breast cancer. But let us hope that the day will come when your daughters, and mine, will find this book, and all others on the topic, "out of print."

Introduction

The diagnosis of breast cancer is a shattering experience. I know. My wife was diagnosed with the disease seventeen years ago. We thought our world would come to an end. My wife struggled with the possibility of losing her life. I was faced with losing the woman I love, and confronted by the prospect of raising two teenagers alone.

Both of us are physicians. She is a pediatrician, and I was an emergency room doctor. We were well-read (at least in medical matters), cool and composed under stress, rational adults able to handle crises—or so we thought. Despite excellent care from breast cancer experts who were also our colleagues and friends, we were totally overwhelmed—by the diagnosis and by the torrent of information that was thrown at us. We had learned about radiation therapy, chemotherapy, and surgery in medical school. Yet we sat there wondering if these people were speaking Greek—or perhaps Latin. It was weeks before we were able to unravel all the details and ramifications, and begin deciding on a course of treatment.

This book, and the video and CD-ROM on which it is based, were created to help you and your loved ones better understand what you are facing, and participate in your treatment and recovery.

The book is a balanced, objective presentation of the latest information, developed in consultation with dozens of top experts in the field, that will help you understand the facts about breast cancer. To this we added candid comments by patients and their partners—the women and men who have "been there," and whose voices can help you understand your own feelings and frustrations at this difficult time.

Facts to Remember About Breast Cancer

- Breast cancer is not a death sentence—98% of those diagnosed are successfully treated if the cancer is detected early.
- Breast cancer can often be treated with breast-conserving surgery—preserving the natural appearance of the breast.
- Excellent options for reconstruction are available if mastectomy is necessary.
- In most cases there is no need to rush your decisions. Take time to learn as much as you can, and to decide what choices are best for you.
- A positive attitude and active participation will improve the outcome of your treatment. Be resolved that you will survive this challenge.

How To Use This Book

The book can be used in conjunction with the *Be A Survivor* ™ DVD or video, where you can actually hear the patient interviews, and see the animated graphics and film clips of the procedures. However, even if you don't have the DVD or the video, the book alone is still an excellent source of information.

Each chapter includes lists of questions you might want to ask your healthcare professionals. For your convenience, these questions are repeated at the end of the book. You can take them, or the whole book, with you on office visits to help you communicate more effectively.

We've tried to lay out the book in a way that mirrors your path through treatment and recovery.

First, we've provided a few suggestions on how to cope with your diagnosis—coming to grips with your feelings so you can think and evaluate the facts. There are tips on how to tell your family, friends, and co-workers about your diagnosis, and how to assemble a network of support to help you get through the tough times.

Next is an overview of breast cancer treatment. If you only read one section in this book, make sure it's this one. It will help you understand how the different aspects of your treatment fit together, and help you evaluate your options.

The majority of the book consists of a detailed description of the various procedures and treatments you may encounter: diagnostic procedures, such as biopsy; surgery, including mastectomy, lumpectomy, and reconstruction techniques; and adjuvant therapies, such as radiation, hormonal therapy, and chemotherapy. We have included information on complementary treatments, such as relaxation, visualization, and acupuncture, which may be valuable additions to your battle with cancer.

The book also will help you make a smooth transition from treatment to recovery, both emotionally and physically. It will show you how to follow-up with your doctor, and how to keep yourself healthy.

The last chapter of the book is devoted to your partner—husband, boyfriend or special man or woman in your life. It not only teaches how to provide support for you, but also speaks directly to the needs of your partner during this time.

At the end of the book we've included several useful reference sections, such as a glossary of important breast cancer terms, a library listing of other books and videos on the subject, and a resource section with names, numbers, and website addresses of organizations and programs that can help you.

We wish you a speedy recovery.

CHAPTER 1

Facing Breast Cancer

"You have breast cancer." These may be the most frightening words you've ever heard. You may feel scared, angry, crushed—or in complete denial. You probably won't remember anything your physician tells you, and will have no idea how to begin dealing with your problem.

First of all, realize that a diagnosis of breast cancer is not a death sentence. Breast cancer is a very treatable disease, and survival rates today are higher than ever before. There are more than one and a half million women who have been handed the same diagnosis many years ago, and are still leading happy, productive lives. My wife Mandy is one of them. She is a sixteen-year survivor, and as strong and active as ever.

The best approach you can take is to resolve, right now, that you will do everything you can to be successful in your battle against breast cancer. This positive attitude will be your best ally.

On the following pages we will discuss the initial steps you need to take to reclaim control over the situation:

- Understand your feelings
- Decide how, when, and with whom to share the news
- Assemble a support network
- Gather the information you need
- Actively participate in planning your treatment.

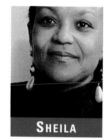

SHEILA

When I heard the doctor say "breast cancer" it was like going underwater. Everything started to move in slow motion, and I couldn't hear anything more. I don't remember how I called my husband, how we drove home. And only when I got to my bedroom, only then I started to cry.

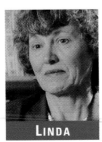

LINDA

Terry was away. He was on a film shoot. And so, I asked a girlfriend to be there when I got home. He called and I had to tell him over the phone. He came home the next day. It was hard.

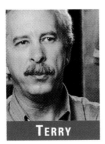

TERRY

I was out of the country on a job and that's when she called and told me that it was malignant. And that was a big blow to both of us. Everything was tossed upside down. I wanted to rush back to her. I didn't really know what it meant to have breast cancer. It could be something that we could get through or it could be a major crisis to her health.

UNDERSTANDING YOUR FEELINGS

Learning that you have breast cancer is an experience that is probably unlike any other in your life. Don't try to suppress the turmoil that you are experiencing. Cry, get angry, shout. Show whatever emotion helps you, because there is no right or wrong response, and you are entitled to feel whatever you are feeling.

The first few weeks after your diagnosis may be the hardest to handle. On some days, questions like "Will I die?" or "Will my husband still love me?" will invade your mind and incapacitate you. On other days, you will be overcome with joy just to hear a single piece of good news. This emotional roller coaster may be difficult to manage, no matter how strong you are. Don't be too hard on yourself if your emotions slip out of your control every once in a while. You don't need to be a superwoman in perfect balance all the time.

Find someone you can talk to about what you are experiencing. This should be a mature, well-adjusted person who can listen without passing judgment. Sometimes very close friends or family members may be too involved in the situation to remain objective. At least initially, it may be best to speak to someone who is more objective, and doesn't have a need to "make it all better."

A good resource for talking about your feelings may be another woman who had breast cancer, or an organized group of breast cancer survivors who meet regularly to offer mutual support, and an opportunity for open communication.

In addition, don't be embarrassed to seek professional help. Group or individual counseling can help you come to grips with your feelings, so you can start on the road to recovery.

SHARING THE NEWS

Communicating With Your Partner

In a misguided attempt to protect your loved one, you may try to hide your emotions from him. Don't. It is far better to involve your partner as soon as possible, so the two of you can find strength in each other, and learn from the beginning how you can work as a team in the weeks and months to come.

Couples may have difficulty adjusting to the role changes that are sometimes necessary. A partner who was responsible for only part of the daily activities may now become the sole breadwinner and homemaker, preparing dinner, changing the bedding and dressings, and providing companionship and emotional support. The sheer weight of these responsibilities can be overwhelming.

A partner's concern or fears also can affect your sexual relationship. Some may worry that physical intimacy will harm the person who has cancer. Others may fear that they might "catch" the cancer or be affected by the drugs. Many of these issues can be cleared up by open communications.

Both you and your partner should feel free to discuss sexual concerns with each other, as well as with your doctor, nurse, or other counselor who can give you the information and the reassurance you need.

Try to remember that your husband, boyfriend or partner probably will be affected by your diagnosis as much as you. In some ways his challenge may be particularly difficult because he will have to manage his own emotions, and at the same time shoulder the task of being your key supporter.

You can help by communicating your needs clearly. "I would love it if you..." will be far better for both of you than some unstated wish left unfulfilled.

Telling Your Children

This is one of the more challenging tasks you and your partner will have to handle. Your first impulse may be to attempt to shield your children from pain by downplaying or withholding information. Don't underestimate their insight. Children's ability to pick up signals is greater than most people realize, and trying to keep a complex situation such as cancer a secret, is practically impossible. More than likely, they will sense that all is not well, and wander away imagining horrors far worse than reality. The next day they will get a dose of misinformation from their classmates, which will only fuel their fears.

A much better approach is a simple and straightforward explanation, geared to each child's age and ability to understand. Conveying the impression that you are comfortable with the situation, and that you trust them, will help them deal with the situation.

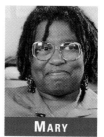

MARY

I was in shock. I couldn't believe it. The last thing I expected to hear was that I had breast cancer. I couldn't have cancer. It was impossible for me to have cancer, because I had all these people to take care of. At my job, I couldn't afford to be sick.

QUESTIONS TO ASK YOUR DOCTOR:

☐ What should I tell my loved ones about my condition?

☐ May I bring members of my family, or a friend, to talk to you directly?

☐ Can you refer me to a counselor or to a support group specializing in breast cancer issues?

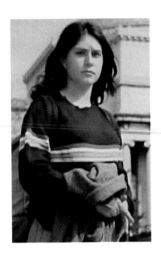

ONE GIRL'S STORY

With the benefit of a sixteen-year hindsight, my wife and I feel that we should have handled our communications with our children better. We "protected" them by presenting a rosy picture. It wasn't until years later that we realized the turmoil that our daughter went through during her Mom's treatment. Here is a school essay she wrote as an eleven-year-old. She didn't show it to us until she went off to college.

My father's face is red. A plate of blackened hamburgers is trembling in his hands. I am looking up at his thick, wrinkled forehead as his mouth opens and closes, spilling angry words: "How could you be so careless? Didn't you realize they were burning?" I do not offer any explanation about my carelessness. I just look down at my sneakers and moan.

There is a deafening crash as my father slams the plate of burned food onto our dining room table. My father, my mother, my teenage brother and I slide noiselessly into our chairs. I can feel hot anger burning at the top of my stomach and shooting up into my throat. I strain to hold back the tears, but the liquid collects on my eyelashes, forming droplets that slowly pull themselves down my cheeks.

"Why are you crying?" My father's voice is louder than he expects it to be. The look on his face tells me that he knows I am not crying over burned hamburgers. He knows exactly why I am crying. He would cry those same frustrated tears if his ego would let him.

I am crying because my mother has cancer. It is the third month of her chemotherapy; the third month we have had to pretend that our family is still as strong as it ever was, that my mother's illness is just a temporary setback.

But tonight I am tired of not being able to be a normal eleven-year-old. I am tired of telling my mother that everything is fine, that she doesn't have to be at my soccer game, that it is OK if she is too sick to eat a piece of my birthday cake. It is no longer fine. Our family cannot survive without my mother. It does not matter that my brother had learned to do laundry while my father goes to PTA meetings and I teach myself how to cook. We cannot bear to think that my mother may die, but we cannot hide the fact that we are thinking it.

"Why are you crying?" My father's words are still reverberating in my brain as I search for a safe place to stare so I do not have to face the sadness in the room. I hear a tiny sound, a low whimper escaping from my mother's side of the table. I glance over at her and watch her hunched shoulders moving rhythmically up and down as she fidgets with the tablecloth. She lifts her pale face and looks around the dining room as if she too is wondering where the sound is coming from. Her eyelids are dark red and tears are slipping effortlessly down her face.

It is the first time I have seen my mother cry. I want to look away, but I keep staring. My mother shakes her head slowly, as if she is scolding herself for revealing the pain she has been harboring underneath her confident exterior.

"Oh God, I'm so sorry." The words come tumbling from my mouth. "I'm so sorry, I'm so sorry." I keep vomiting the words. I run to my mother's side, frantic, hoping I can get to her fast enough to return her to the moment before she began suffering. "I'm sorry, Mommy. I'm sorry." I hug her tighter than I ever have before, letting her hair stick to my wet cheek. "I'm so sorry." The words are not even mine anymore. They are escaping from a place in my body that I never knew existed. I am not thinking about anything else, about what my father and brother must be thinking, about what it will be like after this moment. "I'm sorry..."

I'm sorry that I've been selfish, sorry that I got mad when you weren't excited about my report card, sorry I refused to go with you to your first dose of chemotherapy, sorry that I laughed at your new wig, sorry that I ran away when you threw up in the kitchen sink. I'm sorry I didn't know how you were suffering.

I am holding my mother's trembling body. I rest my chin in the crevasse of her shoulder the way I used to when she knelt down to hug me. The room and its contents no longer exist. My mother and I are alone, clinging to each other, and I am wishing that I could heal her. I press my lips to her ear and whisper, "Mommy, please don't die."

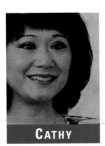

CATHY

I knew that my surgery was just a few days away. And I looked down at my body and at this right breast and I said, "I'm proud of you. You're beautiful. But I am very sorry, you have to go, because you're not my friend anymore." I'm glad I did that. I'm glad that I had made my peace with it.

Dealing with Problems

Cancer is a blow to every family it touches. How you respond to the blow depends on how you have functioned as a family in the past. Families who are used to sharing their feelings with each other usually are able to talk about the disease and the changes it brings. Families in which each member solves problems alone or in which one person has played the major role in making decisions, might have more difficulty coping.

Children, especially, may have difficulty coping with cancer in a parent. Some fear the loss of the parent or begin to imagine their own death. This can play havoc with all aspects of their lives—from school performance, to sleep patterns, to social contacts.

In addition to this upheaval, children often are asked to "play quietly", to perform extra tasks, or to be considerate of others' moods. Some of these demands may far exceed their maturity and understanding.

Tips for better communications with children

- Wait until you and your partner have your emotions under some control—perhaps a day or two after you learn the diagnosis.

- Pick a quiet place and a time when you can talk for as long as necessary, without interruptions.

- Start with a simple statement, adjusted for age and understanding level. For example, "The doctor found a lump in Mommie's breast. It is called cancer, and needs to be taken out..."

- Encourage them to ask questions, and answer them truthfully. Be ready to deal questions that reflect their fear of being abandoned.

- Involve them by assigning tasks that will make them feel like they are contributing to your recovery. This is especially important for younger children, who may feel responsible for your illness.

- You may want to contact a unique organization, Kids Konnected, for information about how to deal with your children's concerns, or to refer them to age-appropriate support groups.

Younger children may resent lost attention. Teenagers can feel torn between expressing independence and a need to remain close to the sick parent. Discipline problems can arise.

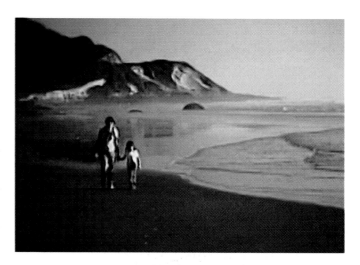

Parents may not have the emotional energy to provide the usual support, love, and authority. It may help if a favorite relative or family friend can devote extra time and attention to the children to help maintain normal family routines as much as possible. Events like trips to the zoo are important, but so is helping with homework, or attending the basketball awards banquet.

In more difficult situations, individual or family counseling can help with the stress. Your physician, a hospital social worker, or hospital psychologist are good sources for referrals to psychologists, psychiatrists, or other mental health professionals trained to counsel individuals and families affected by cancer.

Remember, breast cancer does not need to be a totally negative experience. Instead, it can serve as a tool that will help your family grow stronger and be more united.

Telling Your Family

The people who are close to you also will be affected by your news. They too may need to be angry, cry, and express their emotions. It's a natural part of adjusting to your diagnosis. It will help both you and them to talk openly about each other's feelings. Open communication from the start will go a long way toward strengthening the bonds with your loved ones, and securing the support you'll need.

Sometimes the "extended family" can be just too "extended" or too expressive. Their combined concerns can be overwhelming, and may have a negative effect on you. Feel free to limit the lines of communication with relatives who drain, rather than replenish, your energy. Remember, you are the one in charge, and this is the time when you need unwavering support.

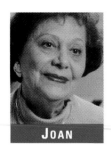

JOAN

When you get that diagnosis, go ahead and cry your eyes out. Cry your eyes out right then, so that you're not bottling up that emotion. It's so terrifying, that for a while you feel as though you're in a fog, and that if you come out of this fog, something terrible is going to happen. So, cry it, vent it, talk it out, and then find out what you can do to help yourself.

Dealing with Friends and Others

Friends can be an excellent source of help and support, particularly if you keep them informed, and help them help you. Some friends will deal well with your illness and will provide gratifying support. Some will be unable to cope with the possibility of your death, and will disappear from your life. Most will want to help, but may be unsure of how to go about it, and will be waiting for clues from you about where to begin.

You may have to be the one who takes the initiative in reestablishing contact. Telephone those who don't call you. Make specific requests for simple things—to run an errand, prepare a meal, come for a visit. No one who is healthy can imagine how much they will be appreciated if they do nothing but pick up a few things off the floor for a woman who may not be able to bend down for a few days after surgery. These small acts bring friends back into contact and help them feel useful and needed.

When it comes to conversational topics, bear in mind that people who don't have experience dealing with cancer may have no idea what is acceptable. "Isn't it too personal to ask about her breast reconstruction?" or "Should I pretend nothing happened?" or "How do I discuss her fears with her, without making things worse?" Help them by being the first to bring up whatever subject you want to discuss.

Beyond the immediate circle of people who are close to you, or who have something positive to offer, telling others about your diagnosis should be on a "need to know" basis. No one is entitled to have information you don't want to give out. Women have gone through entire breast cancer treatments, including surgery, while their co-workers remained unaware of what was going on.

Dealing with Employers

When you return to work, you may encounter discrimination on the grounds that people who have cancer take too many sick days, are poor insurance risks, or will make co-workers uncomfortable.

How can you deal with these issues? Sometimes all it takes is a little education by you. Reassure those concerned that if you do need time off, you will

Find out more about your rights

- Your local American Cancer Society offices have state-specific information about cancer and employment discrimination.

- Your social worker can tell you which state agency is in charge of protecting employee rights.

- Your state's Department of Labor Office of Civil Rights.

- The National Coalition for Cancer Survivorship offers information and limited attorney referrals.

- Regional or national offices of the Civil Liberties Union.

- Your representative's or senator's office has information about Federal and State laws. If you are not sure who represents your district, call your local library.

probably be able to schedule it in advance. Once your treatment is over, you will be able to resume your work as before, and are not likely to have unexpected sick days any more frequently than your co-workers. Explain to everyone that cancer is absolutely not contagious.

Under Federal law, most employers cannot discriminate against disabled workers, including people with cancer. These laws apply to Federal employers, employers that receive Federal funds, and private companies with 25 or more employees. State laws also forbid discrimination based on handicap, but only some protect people with cancer.

If you are applying for a job with a government agency or a firm with government contracts, and believe you did not get the job because of your cancer, you can file a complaint with the Department of Justice.

If you believe you were discriminated against by a private employer because of your cancer, you should file your complaint with the closest regional office of the Equal Employment Opportunities Commission.

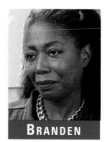

BRANDEN

Develop a really good working relationship with the physicians who are treating you, and let your feelings be known. This is your time. Make sure that everybody is on your team, and don't be afraid to speak up for yourself.

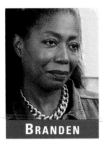

BRANDEN

My cancer was an estrogen positive cancer and I didn't know anything about that term. I went to see the pathologist, and he was very kind. He explained terms like "carcinogenic embryonic antigen." Who has ever heard of stuff like that? He broke it all down, and explained how it fit together. It was very reassuring.

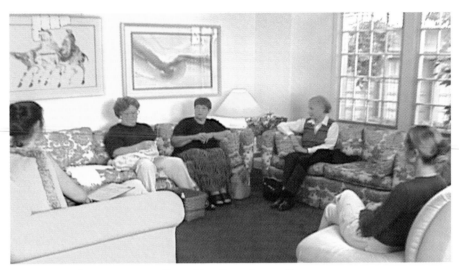

Support groups offer a friendly setting to discuss your concerns.

ASSEMBLING YOUR SUPPORT NETWORK

One of your first steps after your diagnosis should be to establish a network of people who can help you. This network will include your loved ones, your peer support groups, and of course a solid team of healthcare professionals.

Friends and Family

Your loved ones will provide the emotional support and closeness you need, and help you sort out facts and fears.

Try to select one person—your husband, partner, or best friend—who will accompany you when you meet with your doctors or go to your treatments. This companion can help you ask questions, remember information, or write down instructions.

He or she can become the center of your support network, acting as your sounding board, helping you to evaluate information and to make decisions, coordinating support from friends and family, and at times shielding you from excessive attention.

Support Groups

One of the most beneficial things you can do is join a support group. Support groups are groups of people who meet regularly, under the guidance of a trained facilitator, to discuss the participants' concerns.

Programs are organized in a variety of ways. Some groups meet only a few times; others are long-term, enabling members to work through problems. Some are composed of people with the same disease site (for example, breast or colon cancer patients), others by patient age or background. Some are just for patients; others include family or other special people.

Support groups give you a chance to openly discuss your thoughts with others who are going through the same experience. Many hospitals consider some form of group counseling to be part of the standard treatment—as necessary as an exercise class, for example.

Visit the support group a couple of times before joining, so you can be sure that the peer mix meets your needs and expectations.

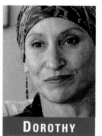

DOROTHY

My group really offers me an opportunity to share my truest feelings, my most private feelings, and my greatest fears in a place where there's support, caring, friendship, and the courage of other people leading you forward.

Your Healthcare Team

Cancer is a complicated disease and no single physician can be an expert in all aspects of the treatment. Developing a treatment plan is a complex task that will involve a number of healthcare professionals—a real team of experts—who will give you their recommendations regarding surgery, chemotherapy and radiation.

Some hospitals and cancer centers already have such teams of breast cancer experts, called multidisciplinary teams. If yours doesn't, the National Cancer Institute, the American Cancer Society, the Susan G. Komen Foundation, or the Y-ME Breast Cancer Organization have resources that will help you find healthcare professionals to add to your team, or to give you a second opinion.

You may want to seek out specialists in specific areas of interest to you, such as chemotherapy or breast reconstruction. Or you may establish a relationship with a generalist who will help you sift through the information you are receiving, or whom you could call with questions that crop up at a time when your regular team is not available.

QUESTIONS TO ASK YOUR DOCTOR:

☐ Could you give me the names of specialists you think I should see?

☐ How about another set of names so I can choose the specialist(s) I like best?

☐ Is there a multidisciplinary breast cancer team in the facility where you practice?

☐ Tell me about your, or your colleagues' experience in dealing with breast cancer.

Here, in alphabetical order, is a list of specialists who may be involved in your treatment:

- **Anesthesiologist:** Administers drugs or gasses which put you to sleep before surgery.

- **Clinical Nurse Specialist:** A nurse with training or knowledge in a specific area, such as post-operative care, chemotherapy, or radiation therapy.

- **Medical Oncologist:** A doctor who administers anti-cancer drugs or chemotherapy.

- **Pathologist:** A doctor who examines the tissue removed during a biopsy, and issues a report to help you and your doctor choose the most effective treatment.

- **Personal Physician:** The doctor who will be responsible for coordinating your treatment. Your personal physician may be a surgeon, radiation oncologist, medical oncologist, or family physician.

- **Physical Therapist:** A specialist who helps with post-surgical rehabilitation using exercise, heat, or massage.

- **Plastic Surgeon:** A doctor specializing in cosmetic surgery, such as breast reconstruction after mastectomy.

- **Radiation Oncologist:** A physician specially trained in using high-energy X-rays for treatment.

- **Radiation Therapy Technologist:** A technologist who works under the direction of the Radiation Oncologist to administer radiation treatment.

- **Social Worker:** A trained professional who can deal with social and economic aspects of treatment, such as helping find a support group or solving an insurance issue.

- **Surgeon:** A doctor specializing in surgery, who will do the initial operation on the cancer.

Getting a Second Opinion

The treatment of your breast cancer is probably the most important issue you will ever face. For your own peace of mind, now and in the future, you may consider getting a second opinion. You are entitled to evaluate all your options, and no competent healthcare provider will object to your listening to another viewpoint.

Changing Doctors

Sometimes you may find that you are not getting along with one of the physicians treating you. The physician may seem abrupt, aloof, and uncaring, or fails to convince you of his competence. If this creates a barrier, let the physician know you wish to see someone else. The physician is probably as aware as you that a relationship based on trust and open communication has not been established, and will be happy to transfer your records to another practitioner.

But remember, a decision to change physicians should be based on reality and not on a quest to find a doctor who will promise a cure, or guarantee to relieve all your fears.

GATHERING INFORMATION

When a woman hears that she has breast cancer, her first response may be a desire to have treatment—any treatment—immediately. But breast cancer is not a medical emergency like a heart attack or an appendicitis. By the time the tumor is found, it may have been growing for years. You can take several weeks to organize your thoughts, gather information, and make a decision about treatment, without jeopardizing the outcome.

Becoming well informed about breast cancer and about your options is one of the most important steps you can take at this stage. Knowledge of the facts will give you a sense of comfort and control.

Studies have shown that a woman's degree of satisfaction with the outcome of her treatment had to do less with the results of the treatment, and more with how much information she had when she made the decision. Take your time to gather all the facts you need, so that you can be comfortable with the decisions that will affect the rest of your life.

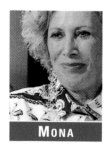

MONA

Too many doctors do not give their patients enough time. If you are not totally content with your physician, go and find somebody who will listen to you, answer your questions, and make you feel you are an important patient. A woman should be assertive and speak up, and if she wants to know why and when and where, she's entitled to these answers.

QUESTIONS TO ASK YOUR DOCTOR:

☐ Can you give me the name of a breast cancer expert who can give me a second opinion?

☐ Could you forward my chart, test results, and my biopsy slides to the doctor who is going to give me a second opinion?

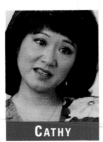

CATHY

Know thy enemy. Know what you're facing and most of your fears will become manageable. That was the most important thing to me—to educate myself about breast cancer.

Your main source of information will be the professionals caring for you. Make lists of topics you want to discuss, and don't hesitate to ask any question, no matter how simple it may seem. Ask your support person to accompany you to the medical appointments, so that you have someone to help you take notes, tape record what was said, or ask additional questions.

Many medical facilities have patient resource centers where you will find collections of books, videos, and CD-ROMs on various aspects of breast cancer treatment.

On a regional or national level, there are several organizations that can be valuable sources of information. They can be found in the Resources section at the end of the book. The specialists at these organizations, many of whom are breast cancer survivors themselves, can answer many general questions about cancer, or send you written materials and information.

A lot of information—and, sadly, misinformation—is readily available on the internet. Be sure that the site you are consulting is sponsored by a reputable organization, and does not represent some individual's bias.

QUESTIONS TO ASK YOUR DOCTOR

☐ Do you, or your clinic or hospital, have a resource center? A library?

☐ Can you refer me to breast cancer groups or organizations in this area?

☐ Where can I find more information about breast cancer?

Government Jobs
You are protected under Section 504 of the Federal Rehabilitation Act of 1973, and by the Americans with Disabilities Act of 1990. Write directly to the agency involved, or contact the Civil Rights Division of the U.S. Department of Justice, Washington, DC. (202) 724-2235.

Private Sector
To obtain the location of your regional Equal Employment Opportunities Commission office and find out exactly what to do, call (800) USA-EEOC.

Overview of Treatment Options

With today's early detection and improved treatment techniques, we can treat breast cancer more successfully than ever before.

The following overview of various therapies will help you understand how and why they are used, alone or in combinations. This information will make it easier for you to understand your physician's recommendations, and arrive at a decision.

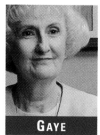

GAYE

I kept a notebook right next to my bed—and whenever I would wake up with a burning question on my mind, I wrote it down. That way when I went to see the doctor, I was better prepared, and I didn't miss anything. It helped me fall asleep faster, too!

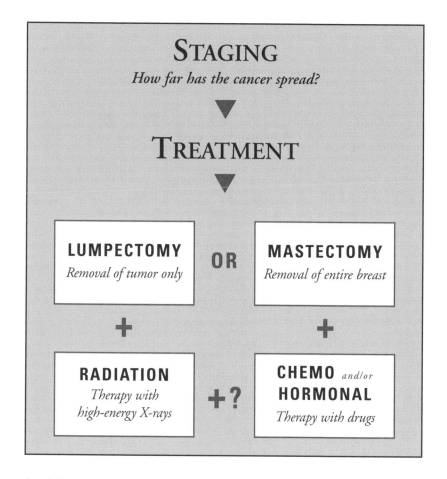

STAGING

How far has the cancer spread?

▼

TREATMENT

▼

LUMPECTOMY	OR	MASTECTOMY
Removal of tumor only		*Removal of entire breast*

+   +

RADIATION	+?	CHEMO *and/or* HORMONAL
Therapy with high-energy X-rays		*Therapy with drugs*

In the following days and weeks, as you explore this book, talk with your healthcare professionals, and gather additional information, you will begin to acquire the knowledge you need to make informed decisions.

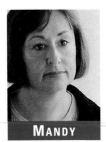

MANDY

Both my husband and I are physicians. We thought we had at least mastered the vocabulary. But after listening to various options for an hour—radiation, brachytherapy, estrogen receptors, nipple reconstruction —we felt completely overwhelmed. It wasn't until the second or third visit that some of it started to make sense.

PLANNING YOUR TREATMENT

Planning your treatment should involve the entire team of specialists who consulted on your case, as well as your partner or your loved ones.

This brief overview was intended to give you a general idea of the treatments available, and of the decision steps involved. Don't worry if you feel confused by the new words and concepts presented here. Most people do at first.

As your case progresses, your team of healthcare professionals will review the information available, and discuss your case with you and among themselves. You'll probably meet with various team members several times, while they develop a recommendation for a course of treatment that's best suited to your case.

The key thing to remember is that it is you who will make the final decision, and all the members of the team need to respect it. That's why it is so important for you to learn all you can about your disease. The more information you can gather before you begin treatment, the better you will feel about your decision, and the more active role you'll be able to take.

CHAPTER 2

Breast Cancer Basics

BREAST ANATOMY AND FUNCTION

First let's review the structure and function of the breast. Some of the terms like "lymph nodes" and "lobules" may be new to you, but they will help you understand breast cancer treatment better.

Although the general shape of a breast is circular or teardrop, breast tissue can be found from the collarbone to the bra line, and from the breastbone to the armpit. That is why it is important for you and your physician to examine that entire area during breast examination.

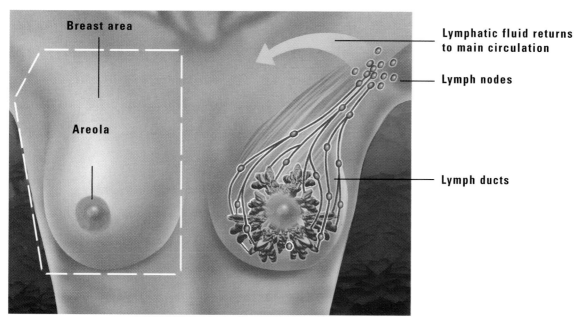

Anatomy of the breast area

MICROSCOPIC VIEWS

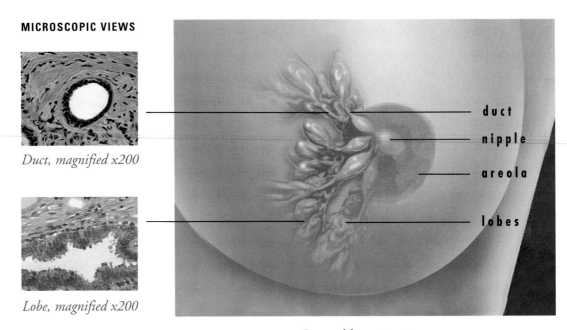

Duct, magnified x200

Lobe, magnified x200

duct

nipple

areola

lobes

Internal breast structures

Breasts are made up of milk-producing glands and milk-carrying ducts, imbedded in fatty tissue and fibrous supportive tissue. The glands are grouped in sections, called lobes. Each lobe has many smaller lobules that end in dozens of tiny grape-like bulbs where milk is produced. Slender tubes called ducts carry the milk from the lobes to the nipple. Most of the rest of the breast is composed of fatty tissue and fibrous supportive tissue.

Two muscles, the pectoralis major and the pectoralis minor, are attached to the ribs under the breast. One of these muscles may be cut to allow room for an implant. There are no muscles within the breast itself.

The area of darker skin around the nipple is called the areola.

Arteries and veins carry blood to and from the breast, supplying it with nutrients and oxygen.

An important concept to understand is the lymphatic system. Lymph is the fluid that leaks out of the blood vessels and accumulates between cells.

Lymph ducts collect this fluid and return it to the main circulation. Along the way, lymphatic fluid is filtered through small bean-shaped structures called lymph nodes, which trap debris such as bacteria, or escaped cancer cells. You may think of the lymphatic system as a network of sewer lines.

Most of the lymphatic fluid from the breast drains toward the armpit area (the axilla), where it is filtered through the axillary lymph nodes. By examining these nodes, the surgeon can get a good indication of whether cancer cells have begun to escape from the breast toward the rest of the body.

How Breasts Grow and Change

From birth to old age, breasts go through more changes than almost any other organ in the body.

One to two years before menarche (first menstrual period) breasts begin to grow under the influence of the female hormones estrogen and progesterone.

During reproductive years, variations in the levels of these hormones cause the breasts to go through monthly cycles: milk glands become engorged and the breasts swell, as if getting ready for a pregnancy, then return to their inactive state again.

At menopause, levels of hormones drop, many milk producing glands shrink and disappear, and some of the breast tissue is replaced with fat.

All these changes sometimes damage the cells' DNA—the genetic material that tells the cell how to divide and grow. This damage may lead to cancer.

WHAT IS BREAST CANCER?

All organs in the body are made of cells. Individual cells are so small, they can be seen only through a microscope. Normally, cells divide in an orderly fashion to replace cells that have aged and died. Controls within each cell tell it to stop dividing if no new cells are needed.

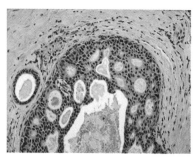

Microscopic view of cancer

Occasionally, damage to DNA during cell duplication may cause the controls to malfunction. Cells begin to divide uncontrollably, forming lumps or tumors.

Tumors

The word "tumor" comes from a Latin word that means "swelling." A tumor could be composed of cells that divide excessively, but that do not invade or damage other parts of the body. A good example is a fibroid in the uterus, or a fibroadenoma in the breast. Both of these are called benign, that is, non-cancerous tumors.

Malignant tumors are composed of aggressively dividing cells that destroy surrounding tissues or travel to other parts of the body. In general conversation, the word "tumor" is often used to refer to a malignant condition, or cancer.

Growth Rate

Growth rate is the speed at which a lump or tumor grows. Different types of breast cancer grow at different rates. The time it takes for a tumor to become twice as large is called doubling time. The average doubling time for most breast cancer tumors is in the range of 50 to 200 days.

The change of the first normal cell into a malignant cell happens years before any evidence of cancer can be detected by any tests that we have today. It may take three to five years for a cluster of cancerous cells to become large enough to be seen on a mammogram. In other words, by the time your cancer has been detected, it has been there for several years. That is why there is no harm in taking a few more weeks to decide on the best treatment possible.

Risk Factors

Who is more likely to get breast cancer? All women are at risk for developing breast cancer. It is the most common cancer in women, with over 200,000 new cases being diagnosed every year. Breast cancer also occurs in men, but rarely.

The main predisposing factor—called risk factor—for breast cancer is age. The older you are, the greater your chances of developing the disease. Four out of five breast cancers are found in women over the age of fifty.

With a positive family history—having a first degree relative such as a mother, sister, or daughter who had breast cancer—a woman's risk of developing breast cancer increases. So women with breast cancer should suggest to their close female relatives that they consult their physicians about their own risk factors, and begin an effective program of early detection.

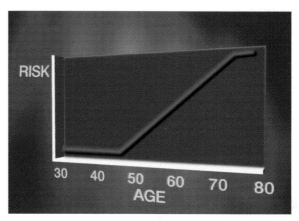

Age is the main risk factor for breast cancer

On the other hand, only about one in twenty cases of breast cancer is truly hereditary—that is, runs in the family—so not having a relative with breast cancer does not reduce the woman's risk.

Some of the other risk factors have a connection to the female hormone estrogen. Interruptions in the levels of this hormone, such as occur during pregnancy and lactation, seem to have a protective effect. In other words, fewer menstrual periods lead to a lower risk. That is probably why women who had one or more children by the age of thirty are at a lower risk, while women who had an early menarche (first menstrual period) or a late menopause (last period) are at a higher risk.

Recent studies indicate that use of certain forms of hormone replacement therapy, or HRT, popular for control of menopause symptoms, may increase a woman's chances of developing breast cancer. Use of low-dose birth control pills has not been linked to breast cancer.

Exercise and a low fat diet may have a protective effect, while alcohol intake of more than one drink per day may increase the risk.

While we don't know exactly what causes breast cancer, we do know that it is not caused by a blow or a physical injury, and that it is definitely not contagious.

Breast Cancer Genes

An important step in understanding breast cancer has been the discovery of the genes that are linked to this disease—BRCA1 and BRCA2.

Genes are specific areas on chromosomes (strands of genetic material contained in our cells) that program the cell with information for growth and function. Scientists found that damage to specific genes on Chromosome 17 correlates with an increased incidence of hereditary-type breast cancer.

There are tests that can detect damage to the BRCA1 and BRCA2 gene. But widespread use of this test to identify women at high risk is being debated because the benefits and consequences of knowing the results are not clear. For example, a "negative" gene test does not mean that the gene is normal. Rather, it indicates that a mutation has not been found. A negative test does not guarantee that the woman will not get breast cancer. Today we can test for two genes, but many more will probably be discovered in the future.

Conversely, a "positive" test does not mean a woman will develop breast cancer, but it does open the door to a variety of problems if the woman's insurance company or employer were to obtain this information.

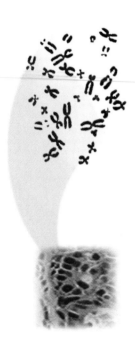

Chromosomes contain genetic information

The best advice for a woman with breast cancer is to suggest to her relatives that they consult a qualified risk counselor before undergoing any genetic testing.

Types of Breast Cancer

Breast cancer types are named according to the part of the breast in which they develop. The most common forms of breast cancer come from cells that line the milk ducts (ductal cancer) or the milk-producing lobules (lobular cancer).

In the early stages, cancer cells divide locally, and do not cross the wall of the duct or lobule. This type of cancer is called *in situ*—meaning "in place." Once the cancer cells cross the lining of the duct or lobule, they are called *infiltrating*, or *invasive*. Do not be unduly alarmed if you are told your cancer is "invasive." Most cancers are, so your invasive cancer is the "normal" cancer.

Today about one in five cases of diagnosed breast cancers fall into the non-invasive, or in situ category—either *ductal carcinoma in situ* (DCIS), or *lobular carcinoma in situ* (LCIS).

DCIS cancers are highly curable. Some physicians don't even refer to them as cancer, but rather as "precancerous lesions," since DCIS may never progress to be an invasive cancer.

The treatment of DCIS may not follow the same plan as for invasive cancers, so we have dedicated a separate chapter to this non-invasive form of the disease. You still need to read the chapters on staging, surgery and radiation to understand the principles involved.

LCIS is a non-invasive growth that is not considered cancerous, but women who are diagnosed with LCIS have about a 1% per year risk of developing invasive breast cancer. That means that twenty years after diagnosis, the risk is about 18%. What is important to know is that the invasive cancer can occur in either breast, and not necessarily where the LCIS was originally found. In other words, LCIS is not a precursor, but a marker.

Infiltrating or invasive cancers, where malignant cells cross the lining of the duct or lobule, are more advanced than in situ cancers. They invade, or infiltrate, adjacent tissues. The most common type of breast cancer is the infiltrating ductal carcinoma. More than half of all cases are of this type.

Other types of breast cancer are less common. One example is *Paget's Disease*, a cancerous growth that first appears as scaling on the nipple, and may be confused for a simple rash. Another is *inflammatory cancer*, a rare form of cancer that grows quickly, causing redness and swelling of the breast. This is really the only form of breast cancer in which the treatment decision needs to be made as soon as possible.

How Cancer Spreads

As a malignant tumor grows, it may spread locally, invading and sometimes destroying other tissues, or cells may break away from the tumor and get into the lymphatic vessels, or into the blood vessels, and travel to dis-

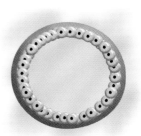

Normal duct

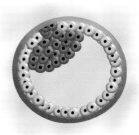

In situ cancer

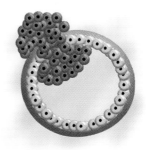

Invasive cancer

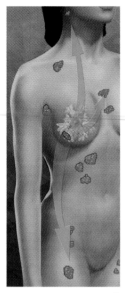

Breast cancer spread

tant parts of the body. Some of the breakaway cells will be trapped in the lymph nodes of the armpit, or axilla. Examination of these nodes by a procedure called axillary lymph node dissection, can help determine the stage (the degree of spread) of the cancer.

If cancer cells escape beyond the lymph nodes, or enter the circulatory system directly, they can spread to the liver, brain, lungs, and bones, forming new tumors called *metastases*. These distant metastases are the most worrisome, because they can damage vital organs. This advanced stage of breast cancer, called *metastatic* cancer, is less common and its management is more difficult.

To make sure that no cancer cells remain anywhere in the body, it is often necessary to use *systemic therapy*—therapy that reaches all the organs, in all parts of the body, by means of the blood stream. This is explained in the Chemotherapy and Hormone Therapy chapters.

CHAPTER 3

Diagnosis & Staging

The only sure way to confirm a diagnosis of breast cancer is to perform a biopsy—that is, to remove a small piece of the tumor, and have it examined under a microscope by a pathologist—a specialist in tumor identification.

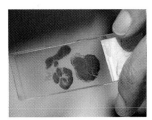

Tumor sample ready for examination under a microscope

The sample can be obtained either with a needle, or surgically. Odds are that if you are reading this book, you already may have had a biopsy that showed your tumor was malignant. If so, feel free to skip to the Staging section on page 36.

DIAGNOSIS

Biopsy

If the tumor is small, or if there is a good possibility that it is not cancerous, your physician may choose either a fine needle aspiration or a core needle biopsy.

Fine Needle Aspiration

Fine Needle Aspiration, or FNA, is done with a very thin needle connected to a syringe. The needle is moved in and out several times to obtain the best sample possible. It feels like having your blood drawn, and does not require a local anesthetic.

The material drawn into the syringe will be sent to a pathologist for analysis. Even if no cancer cells are found, your doctor may want to have the lump removed surgically.

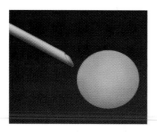

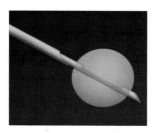

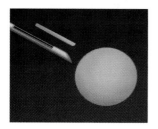

Core needle taking
a biopsy sample

Core Needle Biopsy

Core Needle Biopsy is done with a larger needle, which can yield a larger sample. The procedure can be done under a local anesthetic and takes only a few minutes. It is the least invasive form of biopsy, but it does require the expertise of a specialist. Most women who have had the procedure report only minor discomfort.

The core biopsy is performed with a device that works like an ear-piercing instrument: it propels a needle very rapidly through the lesion. A special notch in the needle traps a sliver of tissue for examination. Samples obtained with core biopsy are large enough to be cut into thin slices and examined under the microscope, providing a diagnosis that some doctors feel is more reliable than that from a FNA.

Several newer devices use a small rotating cutter and vacuum to remove an even larger sample.

Whatever device is used, if the lesion is non-palpable (in other words, cannot be felt by hand) the needle is guided using special mammography equipment, called a stereotactic unit. This equipment enables the radiologist to place the needle precisely into the tumor, even if it is as small as a pea. The needle can also be guided with the help of a hand-held ultrasound unit.

The biopsy also can be done using ultrasound equipment, or a special MRI scanner, to guide the needle. The choice generally depends on what your physician is most comfortable with.

Surgical Biopsy

Another way your doctor may choose to obtain a biopsy is surgically. A surgical biopsy is performed under local anesthesia, sometimes with sedation. Most surgical biopsies are excisional, in other words the surgeon removes (excises) the entire tumor.

The surgical biopsy takes about an hour, and causes minimal post-operative pain that goes away in a few days. You can usually begin doing non-strenuous work the day after the biopsy, although you should not lift heavy objects for a few weeks. The incision usually heals within ten days. You should avoid activities that bounce your breast, such as jogging.

TUMOR TESTING

The sample of tumor will be examined under a microscope by a pathologist, who will identify the cells and determine whether the tumor is benign or malignant.

If the tumor is malignant, additional tests may be performed to help your physician determine the type of treatment that will be most effective.

Estrogen Receptors and Progesterone Receptors

One of the most common tests is for estrogen and progesterone receptors. Receptors are areas on the surface of cells to which substances, such as the hormones estrogen and progesterone, can bind—much like a lock accepts a key. When the hormone binds to its receptor, it activates the cell, making it divide.

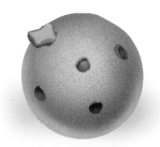

Estrogen binding to receptor site

If a tumor is composed of cells that have estrogen or progesterone receptors, it is called estrogen receptor (ER) positive, or progesterone receptor positive, or hormone receptor positive. The results of this tests are important, because ER positive tumors can be treated with drugs that block the action of the hormones. Tumors lacking estrogen and progesterone receptors usually cannot be treated with this class of drugs.

HER-2/neu (c-erb B2)

An oncogene is a gene which when turned on, leads to development of a cancer. Women with an abnormally high level of an oncogene called HER-2/neu tend to develop much more aggressive breast cancers. A test will determine your level of HER-2/neu and help your oncologist decide if you are a good candidate for treatment with a drug called Herceptin.

OTHER TUMOR TESTING

There are other factors which are currently being evaluated and may help determine the tumor's response.

Growth rate

When cells divide, they go through a number of specific steps, or phases. S-phase is the phase of the cell cycle in which DNA is replicating—making copies of itself, so that a complete set will go to each new cell. Having a high percentage of cells in the S-phase indicates more rapid tumor growth, and a tumor that is more dangerous.

Ploidy

Genes are clusters of DNA that are strung together in long strands called chromosomes, and form the "blue-prints" that determine what a cell does and how it works. Cells having an abnormal number of chromosomes (or an abnormal amount of DNA) are called aneuploid and may indicate a somewhat worse prognosis.

p53

A suppressor gene is a gene which protects the body against cancer. If this gene is mutated (damaged), its protective effect may be lost. Mutated p53 can be detected in the cells of some breast cancers and is associated with a poorer prognosis.

Vascular or lymphatic invasion

One of the factors to consider in anticipating how aggressive a tumor will be, is the tumor's ability to develop its own system of blood vessels to help it grow—angiogenesis. Microscopic examination can show if the tumor is invading lymph ducts or blood vessels, which would indicate a worse prognosis.

Genetic profiling

Newly-developed, still experimental tests can evaluate a large number of genes in a tumor tissue sample. Studies are underway to attempt to determine which sets of genes can predict whether a particular tumor will respond to a specific treatment.

THE PATHOLOGY REPORT

If you had a fine needle aspiration, the pathologist may be able to identify the general type of cancer and report within an hour of the biopsy. For a more complete identification of the cells, a larger sample, such as from a core needle biopsy or surgical biopsy, is required. This report will generally take several days.

The final pathology report can only be issued after the tumor is removed during surgery. This report will specify the size of the tumor, the type of cell the tumor is composed of, and whether there is tumor spread to lymph nodes. This information is essential for planning your treatment.

ADDITIONAL TESTS

Why more tests? A biopsy can confirm that the diagnosis is cancer, but it will not show whether the cancer has spread to other parts of the body. This information is important to determine the stage of the tumor.

To determine this, additional tests may need to be performed, including chest X-rays, blood tests, CAT scans or MRIs of the abdomen or other parts of the body, and bone scans. The surgeon may also remove lymph nodes from your axilla to check them for cancer spread, although this is generally done at the time that you have your surgery.

CT Scan

CAT scan, CT scan, or Computerized Axial Tomography all mean the same thing. This test uses ordinary X-rays, and a rotating film/source system to obtain detailed images of your body. The test is short and painless.

MRI

MRI or Magnetic Resonance Imaging uses a combination of magnetic energy and ordinary radio waves to create images of the inside of your body.

Because the MRI unit can feel cramped, notify the technologist or your physician if you feel uncomfortable in confined spaces. MRI is painless, and does not expose you to X-ray radiation. The test takes about an hour.

Bone Scan

Some of the more common sites to which breast cancer cells may metastasize, or spread, include bones. The most effective way to find these metastases is to perform a nuclear scan. This test is generally done if the tumor is large, or the lymph nodes are positive and there is a good chance that tumor cells may be found in other areas of the body.

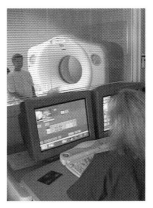

Preparing for a CT scan

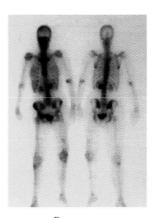

Bone scan

For this scan, tiny amounts of radioactive substance are injected into a vein. Once inside the body, the radioactive substance concentrates in areas where there is an unusually increased number of blood vessels—a "hot spot"—that may correspond to a new growth of cancer cells.

PET Scan

The PET scan is a newer addition to cancer staging tests. It works on a principle similar to the bone scan.

TUMORS, ACTUAL SIZE

1 cm

2 cm

HOW STAGE IS DETERMINED

Each cancer is unique, each woman is different, and the combination of treatment options is practically endless. To help determine who should get what treatment, cancer specialists rely on staging—a system that places the cancer into a certain group. The stage of your tumor is the most important factor in deciding what type of treatment is best for you.

TNM

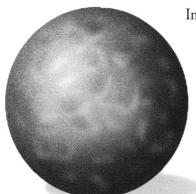

In simplified form, staging is based on: the size of the tumor; presence of cancer cells in the lymph nodes; and metastasis, or spread, to other organs. This is the so called TNM—tumor, node, metastasis—staging system.

Tumor size is determined when the tumor is removed and sent to the pathologist.

Lymph nodes are checked for evidence of tumor spread at the time of surgery in a procedure called axillary lymph node dissection.

5 cm

Metastasis, or spread to other organs, is assessed with bone scans, X-rays, CAT scans, and blood tests. Putting all this information together is called *staging.*

STAGES OF BREAST CANCER

There are several staging systems in use. Here is one of them:

Stage 0 (in situ):

Ductal or Lobular carcinoma in situ, or Paget's Disease of the nipple.

Stage I:

Tumor is 2 cm (3/4 inch) or smaller. Axillary lymph nodes are negative and there is no evidence of distant metastases.

Stage II:

Tumor is 2-5 cm in size (about 3/4 to 2 inches). Axillary lymph nodes may or may not be positive for cancer. Even if the tumor is smaller than 2 cm, but the lymph nodes are positive, cancer is also considered Stage II.

Stage III:

Tumor is larger than 5 cm (2 inches) and axillary lymph nodes are positive. Tumor may extend into the pectoral muscles or into the skin of the breast, but there are no distant metastases.

Stage IV:

If metastasis to other organs has occurred, cancer is considered Stage IV regardless of the size of the tumor, or the number of positive axillary lymph nodes.

You may find it helpful to think of stage as degree of risk presented by a particular tumor.

At one end of the scale are the low-risk situations: very tiny tumors that have not spread to lymph nodes, and that are composed of cells that are not very aggressive.

Further along are slightly larger tumors, still smaller than about a half inch (1 cm), still without evidence of lymph node spread, but often more aggressive.

At the other end of the scale are the situations that involve the greatest risk: larger tumors that have invaded the lymph nodes.

If you are at the low-risk end of the scale, your treatment may require breast conserving surgical removal of the tumor plus a course of radiation therapy, and perhaps a less aggressive form of hormonal therapy or chemotherapy.

Larger tumors may be treated with more aggressive chemotherapy.

For high-risk tumors, at the far end of the scale, there are a wide variety of options, ranging from combination chemotherapy to dose dense chemotherapy.

Surgery

To ensure the best chance for successful treatment of breast cancer, it is important to remove all the cancerous tissue, using the most direct approach possible. This means some type of surgery. Other treatments, such as radiation therapy, chemotherapy, or hormonal therapy cannot replace surgery, but do play a very important role later in the treatment process.

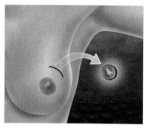

Lumpectomy: removal of the tumor with a margin of healthy tissue.

There are two surgical options: One is to remove just the tumor, with a safety margin of healthy breast tissue around it, conserving most of the breast. This is called wide local excision, partial mastectomy, or lumpectomy. This breast-conserving surgery is usually followed by radiation therapy—treatment of the breast area with high energy X-rays to destroy any cancer cells that may have remained behind.

The other option is to remove the entire breast in a procedure that is called a mastectomy. In the past, women dreaded this operation almost as much as the cancer itself. But the mastectomy techniques used today are much less disfiguring than the ones used years ago, and offer excellent possibilities for cosmetic reconstruction.

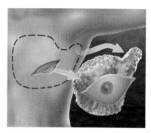

Mastectomy: removal of the entire breast.

Many studies have now proven that breast-conserving therapy is as effective as a mastectomy. The choice depends on the type, size, and degree of spread of your tumor, and on your personal preference. Many women do not realize that they can choose between lumpectomy and mastectomy, without compromising the treatment outcome, how long they will live, or their chance of a recurrence.

We will review the pros and cons as we describe each procedure. Then, in consultation with your healthcare team, and armed with an open mind, you can pick the procedure that is best for you.

Chapter 4

Lumpectomy

What is a Lumpectomy?

If the tumor is small and confined to a single location in the breast, you may have the option of having breast-conserving surgery. The goal of this rela-

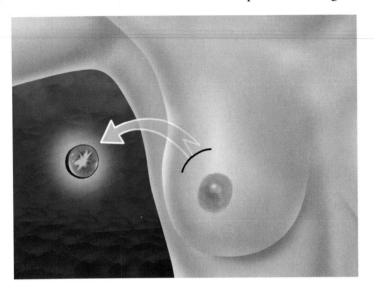

tively simple procedure is to remove the whole tumor, while conserving as much breast tissue as possible. A margin of normal breast tissue is also removed to make sure no malignant cells are left behind.

The technical term for this type of surgery is partial mastectomy. Most people commonly refer to it as a lumpectomy—a "lump-removal", so to speak. Depending on how much breast tissue is removed, the procedure may also be called wide excision, segmental mastectomy, or quadrantectomy. The specific technique used may vary from surgeon to surgeon and from case to case.

The cosmetic result of breast conserving surgery will vary with the location and size of the tumor, and the size of the breast. Removing a large tumor from a large breast may result in a normal-looking breast, but removing even a small tumor from a small breast may lead to noticeable change in breast size and shape that may be cosmetically significant.

Very large tumors may be treated first with chemotherapy (this is called neoadjuvant chemotherapy), in order to shrink them before removing them surgically. Currently there are new techniques that are being tested that would allow the physician to destroy a small tumor without surgery. These so-called ablation techniques rely on laser beams, or heated or cooled needles placed directly into the tumor to destroy the cells.

Breast conserving surgery almost always requires additional treatment of the breast area with high energy X-rays (radiation therapy) to kill any surviving cancer cells that might be left behind.

Questions to Ask Your Surgeon:

- [ ] Is lumpectomy an option for me? Why or why not?

- [ ] How will my breast look after the treatment? Can you show me pictures?

- [ ] How much pain should I expect in the first few days?

- [ ] How long before I can go back to my regular activities?

Before Surgery

A lumpectomy may be done in a hospital operating room, or in an outpatient surgery center. You may be able to go home the same day. You will want to have a friend or relative accompany you to the hospital, to provide moral support, to meet you after surgery, and to drive you home.

You'll probably be instructed not to eat or drink after midnight on the night before surgery.

If your tumor was found on a mammogram, but is difficult or impossible to feel by touch, your surgeon may request that a needle localization procedure be done before you go to surgery. For this procedure, a radiologist will use a special mammography unit to pinpoint the location of the tumor, then mark it by inserting a thin wire into the breast. The surgeon will follow this wire to find the tumor more easily during surgery.

Before the surgery you'll meet with the anesthesiologist to decide whether you'll have general or local anesthesia. The choice depends on your health and on your personal preferences.

You'll also be asked to sign an informed consent form as an indication that you understand the procedure and the possible complications, such as infection and bleeding. Make sure to read the form carefully and ask for explanations of any parts that you are not comfortable with.

The Surgical Procedure

A lumpectomy takes about an hour. The surgeon will make a skin incision over the tumor area and remove the tumor with a small amount of surrounding healthy breast tissue. This margin, about one-half to three-quarters of an inch in thickness, helps decrease the chance that any tumor cells are left behind.

The surgical specimen will be sent to a pathologist who will examine it under a microscope and determine whether the margins were clear of tumor cells. If tumor cells are found along the edges, it means that some cancerous cells may have been left behind. Another lumpectomy may be done to get clear margins. In some cases, a mastectomy may be required.

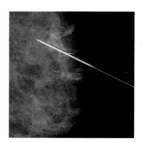

Breast needle localization X-ray

QUESTIONS TO ASK YOUR ANESTHESIOLOGIST:

☐ If I have general anesthesia, how long will it take me to get back to normal?

☐ What will I feel and hear if I have local anesthesia?

☐ Will you give me something to control the pain after I wake up from the anesthetic?

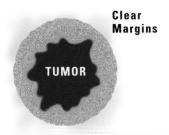

Clear Margins

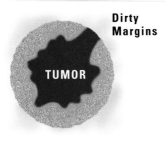

Dirty Margins

Margins are checked for tumor spread

Recovery after Lumpectomy

After the lumpectomy, you'll be taken to the recovery room for a short while, and then discharged to go home. If you didn't have an axillary lymph node dissection at the same time as the lumpectomy, you'll be able to resume normal activities almost immediately.

Follow the aftercare instructions you receive regarding how long to keep the incision dry, when to return for a follow-up visit to your surgeon, and when to have the sutures removed.

Radiation Therapy

An important part of breast conserving treatment is radiation therapy. Radiation therapy uses high energy X-rays applied to the breast area to kill any possible remaining cancer cells.

This can be done either with a special machine, which involves treatments five days a week for five to eight weeks at a special facility, or with special radioactive seeds, which only takes one to three days, and irradiates only part of the breast, or with various other techniques of accelerated partial breast radiation.

You can learn more about the different options for radiation therapy in Chapter 6.

Is Lumpectomy Right for Me?

What is better, mastectomy or lumpectomy? Numerous research studies, involving thousands of women and many years of follow-up, show that there is no difference in survival between the two procedures. Despite these very conclusive studies, some physicians may still recommend a mastectomy, due to personal bias. If your doctor does not offer you a lumpectomy as an option, make sure you understand why.

Besides being equally effective, breast conserving surgery offers several advantages over a mastectomy. You keep your breast, (although you may notice a change in shape), and you avoid the emotional trauma of losing the breast. A good cosmetic result can be expected, and sensation in the nipple and skin area can usually be preserved.

However, not all women can have breast conserving surgery. If the tumor is large, or the breast is small, the cosmetic results may not be acceptable after the tumor is removed. Some women are unable or unwilling to undergo the course of radiation therapy required after a lumpectomy. And a few prefer the peace of mind they expect after a mastectomy.

To ensure that you are receiving the best treatment possible for your particular case, you must meet certain criteria that will make you a good candidate for breast conserving surgery.

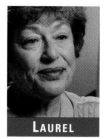

LAUREL

I had a lumpectomy with a local anesthetic. It was extremely easy and when it was over I felt physically very good. I was able to go home with relatively little pain.

A lumpectomy would not be recommended in the following situations:

- There is more than one tumor in the breast.

- The tumor is so big or the breast so small that the cosmetic result would not be satisfactory after removal of the tumor.

- The tumor was found to extend beyond the margins of the tissue removed during initial surgery.

- You are not willing to have radiation therapy, or there is no convenient radiation therapy facility near you.

- You prefer to have a mastectomy.

ADVANTAGES OF LUMPECTOMY:

- breast is spared

- preserves normal nipple and skin sensation

- yields good cosmetic results

It is important to remember that no decision needs to be made overnight. You can take up to several weeks to gather information. You do not need to make the decision alone. Consult your healthcare professionals, consider getting a second opinion, and talk things over with your loved ones.

Susan G. Komen Foundation, the American Cancer Society's Reach to Recovery program, WIN-ABC's Breast Buddy program, and the Y-Me Breast Cancer Organization will be happy to discuss your choice with you and put you in touch with other women who had the same type of surgery.

See the Resources section for information on contacting these organizations.

MASTECTOMY

What is a Mastectomy?

The other option for surgical treatment of breast cancer is mastectomy. Mastectomy, or surgical removal of the breast, has been used to treat breast cancer for several centuries.

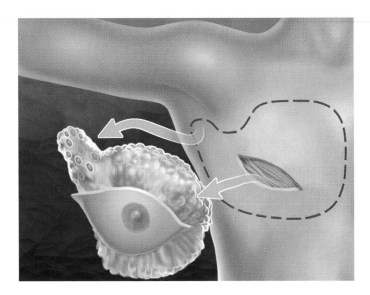

The radical mastectomy, which removed the entire breast, the lymph nodes in the armpit, and one of the major muscles of the chest wall, was based on the mistaken belief that the more tissue removed, the better the chances of curing the cancer. This procedure caused so much deformity, that women feared it as much as the cancer itself.

In the 1970s and 1980s, research proved that there was no advantage in removing the chest muscles, and the modified radical mastectomy, which spares these muscles yielding a more cosmetically acceptable result, was introduced. Now the radical mastectomy is almost never used.

QUESTIONS TO ASK YOUR ANESTHESIOLOGIST:

☐ Will you give me something to help me relax before surgery?

☐ How long will it take me to get back to normal after a general anesthetic?

☐ What are the side effects of anesthesia?

The modified radical mastectomy performed today removes as much of the breast tissue as possible, including the nipple and the areola, and a number of axillary lymph nodes, but not the muscles. Patients can choose from a variety of reconstruction techniques that offer pleasing cosmetic results.

The current trend that strives to preserve as much of the breast as possible has lead to the development of the so-called *skin-sparing mastectomy*. In this procedure the incision includes only the nipple, a narrow margin of skin around it, and the skin directly over the cancer, leaving most of the breast skin intact. This type of mastectomy makes it easier to have a single-stage reconstruction.

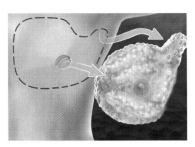

Skin-sparing mastectomy

Before Surgery

A mastectomy is generally done in a hospital, under general anesthesia. After a date is set, someone on your surgeon's staff will review with you the admission process for the particular hospital where the operation will take place.

Ask someone in the surgeon's or hospital's business office whether your insurance covers surgical fees, hospital room, anesthesiologist's fees, and other charges. Make a list of all the medications you are taking, both prescription and over-the-counter, since some of them may have adverse effects during anesthesia or surgery. (For example, aspirin-containing preparations can increase bleeding.) Some medications may need to be discontinued weeks before surgery.

Pack all the personal belongings you may need: a nightgown, slippers, toiletries, books or an iPod, perhaps a favorite pillow, and a change of loose clothing to wear when you go home.

Most people undergoing surgery enjoy having a friend or relative accompany them to the hospital and meet them after the procedure. If you are going to be sent home the same day, you will definitely need someone to drive you.

You'll be instructed not to eat or drink anything after midnight on the night before the surgery.

On the day of the surgery, you'll first go through an admission process at the hospital. Your surgeon already will have reviewed with you all aspects of the procedure, and the possible risks and complications. On the day of admission, the hospital staff will ask you to sign an informed consent form listing your doctor's name and the name of the surgical procedure you are having.

The form requires that you verify the following:

- That the risks of the surgery and the anesthetic have been explained to you.

- That intravenous medication, including drugs, anesthesia, and blood transfusions, may be administered.

THINGS TO TAKE WITH YOU TO THE HOSPITAL:

- nightgown
- slippers
- toiletries
- books
- iPod
- favorite pillow
- change of loose clothing for going home

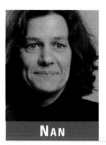

NAN

I think my lover's mastectomy scar was easier to look at than looking at the biopsy scar. The mastectomy scar, even though it was much more traumatic, was very clean. So to me, it wasn't terribly shocking, and there was a sense of relief in it.

- That any tissue removed during the surgery may be examined and disposed.

- That you understand all of the foregoing and that you consent to the surgery.

Make sure you feel comfortable with what you are signing. Cross out and initial anything you don't agree to. If there is anything on the form that worries you, ask to see your doctor.

Blood transfusions are rarely needed during lumpectomies or mastectomies, but may be required for certain types of breast reconstruction. Many people are concerned about contamination of banked blood with HIV, the virus that causes AIDS.

You may wish to discuss with your physician the possibility of donating and storing your own blood before your surgery so that it can be used, should you need it. You will need to donate the blood at least one week before surgery.

An anesthesiologist or a nurse anesthetist will meet with you and select a general anesthetic that is best suited to your medical condition.

They need to know about:

- Your medical history and any problems with your heart, lungs, circulation.

- Any current conditions such as skin infections, colds, or tooth decay.

- Any allergies.

- Any prescriptions, over-the-counter medications, or drugs that you may be taking

- Your smoking and drinking patterns.

The Surgical Procedure

The anesthesiologist will meet you in the staging area, start an intravenous line (an "IV") in one of your arms using a small needle, and perhaps give you something to help you relax.

When the surgical team is ready, you will be taken to the operating room. Several devices will be attached to you, such as an automatic blood pressure cuff, a heart monitor, and a blood oxygen monitor. The anesthesiologist will inject a drug into your vein through the tubing, and you will fall asleep almost

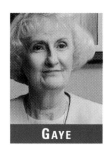

GAYE

I was not happy about having to deal with drains. The nurse showed me how to use them, and I said, "I don't think I can do this." But I did, and my husband helped me. He was right there with everything that we did.

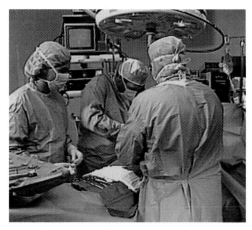

Surgeons performing a mastectomy

immediately. A tube may be placed through your mouth to maintain a way for you to breathe during the surgery. Your blood pressure, pulse, and breathing will be closely monitored during the entire procedure.

The total mastectomy takes two to three hours. Breast tissue extends from the collar bone to the edge of the ribs, and from the breast bone to the muscles in the back of the armpit. The surgeon will make an incision, then remove as much of the breast tissue as possible.

The tissue will be sent to the pathologist, who will examine it for any evidence of cancer spread beyond the breast.

You may also undergo a procedure called an axillary lymph node dissection—removal of a number of lymph nodes, or a few sample nodes from your armpit for examination by the pathologist. Presence or absence of cancer cells in these lymph nodes will help determine your future treatments. If your tumor was very small, or if the pathologist's report said that it was non-invasive (DCIS), then you may not have an axillary lymph node dissection.

You will find more information about this procedure in the section on axillary lymph node dissection later in this chapter.

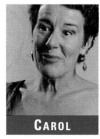

CAROL

I have a very clear memory of the first time I took the bandages off. I literally went crazy. All of a sudden it was in my face. That breast wasn't there anymore. And it wouldn't ever be there.

When the procedure (mastectomy or node dissection) is completed, one or two tubes called *drains* will be placed under the skin to help remove the fluid that accumulates at the site of surgery. If you go home with the drains, you'll receive instructions on how to care for them. You'll be shown how to empty the suction bulbs attached to the drains and keep a record of the volume and color of the fluid removed. The drains will be removed at a follow-up visit to your surgeon, or as soon as the drainage decreases.

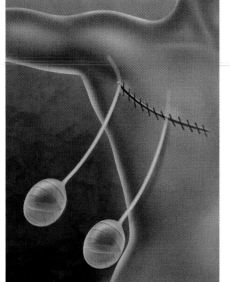
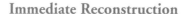

Drains

Immediate Reconstruction

If you've decided to have immediate reconstruction of the breast, the plastic surgeon will take over while you are still asleep. Reconstruction can be done using your own tissues—from the abdomen, back, or buttocks—or using a synthetic implant. The procedure may take anywhere from an hour to six or eight hours, depending on the method used.

You can learn about reconstruction options in more detail in Chapter 5.

Recovery after Mastectomy

After surgery, you'll be taken to the recovery room. As you wake up from the anesthetic, you may feel cold, and your throat may be sore from the tube used for anesthesia. You may fade between waking and sleeping for several hours.

Whatever surgery they are going to have, most women like to have a friend or relative meet them after the operation. You can ask your surgeon how long it will take before you will be brought to your room after surgery and to arrange with the hospital to allow that person to meet you there.

Most women will stay in the hospital for one or two nights after a mastectomy, and somewhat longer after a mastectomy with reconstruction.

Each woman reacts to surgery differently. Most can take a short walk in and out of their hospital room the day of surgery. The next day, most are able to eat a regular diet and get around.

Recovering at Home

Once you're home, you'll probably feel more tired than usual for a while. Don't be discouraged. You've just been through general anesthesia and major surgery, and fatigue is to be expected.

Take sponge baths for a few days after surgery until your incision starts to heal. Don't shower until your drains are removed, and the surgeon tells you that it is alright to get the incision wet. When you do shower, treat the skin gently and pat, rather than rub, the incision.

Immediately after surgery, you'll probably have trouble moving your arm due to muscle tightness and soreness around the shoulder. Use the arm as tolerated immediately after surgery, but avoid active stretching or pulling until the drains are removed and you get your doctor's approval. Don't be afraid to enlist the help of a friend or relative until your arm function returns.

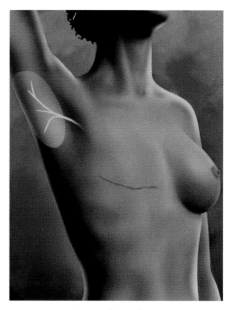

Area of numbness

Many women return to work as soon as they feel better, even while their chemotherapy and radiation treatments are continuing. If your job requires lifting or strenuous physical activity, you may need to change your activities until you have fully regained your strength.

Possible Side Effects

If you had an axillary lymph node dissection you may experience numbness in the upper inner arm and armpit area, caused by injury to one of the nerves. If this happens to you, you may need to be particularly careful when you shave your underarm. The numbness will usually improve over months or years, but the sensation may never be completely normal.

Another side effect of axillary lymph node dissection is swelling of the arm, called lymphedema, which is caused by scarring around lymphatic ducts injured during surgery, or as a result of radiation therapy.

You can learn more about lymphedema later in this chapter.

QUESTIONS TO ASK YOUR SURGEON:

☐ How much pain should I expect in the first few days after the procedure?

☐ What can I do to relieve the pain?

☐ Do I need to arrange to have someone help me with my daily activities?

☐ How long before I can go back to my regular work or leisure activities?

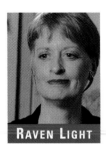

RAVEN LIGHT

For me, to this day, I have a hard time looking in my bedroom mirror at the scar. The scar is a very good, very neat scar, but I'm always petrified that maybe I'll see new, cancerous lumps on either side.

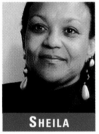

SHEILA

The clusters of cancerous cells were scattered throughout the breast, making lumpectomy not a choice. Because if they removed enough tissue the breast would be totally misshapen, and there would also be the possibility of cancer cells left behind.

Exercises After Mastectomy

The goal of exercising is to regain the full range of motion in your shoulder and arm as soon as possible. But don't attempt to begin exercising without specific instructions from your healthcare provider.

Exercises must be done in stages. After the drains are removed, your doctor or physical therapist may assign pendulum-like movements with your arm, to begin loosening any tightness in the shoulder area.

- Holding on to something for support (such as a chair or desk), lean forward at the waist and swing your arm in gradually enlarging circles. Make ten circles, rest, then repeat in the other direction.

After the sutures are removed, you may be told to begin stretching exercises to regain full motion in the shoulder.

- Walk your fingers up the wall, until you feel mild pain in the incision, and note how far you can reach each day.
- Throw a rope or an old tie over a door, and move your arms up and down in a see-saw motion.
- Walk your arm up your back as far as you can.

Many communities offer swimming, exercise, and dance classes specifically for breast cancer patients. The YWCA Encore program is one of them. Check the Resources section for other suggestions.

Is Mastectomy Right for Me?

Numerous research studies, involving thousands of women and many years of follow-up, show that there is no difference in survival in patients treated with lumpectomy and radiation, or with mastectomy.

There is a slightly higher rate of local cancer recurrence (in the breast area itself) following lumpectomy: one out of a hundred women treated with lumpectomy will develop a local recurrence within a year. (In other words, there is a 1% per year recurrence rate. The chance of having a recurrence within ten years is 10%.) Local recurrences are not life threatening, and can be controlled by performing a mastectomy.

Since there is no difference in numbers of life-threatening distant metastases (cancer in other sites in the body) between lumpectomy and mastectomy, there is no difference in life expectancy between the two procedures.

So the choice is between running a slightly higher risk of a local recurrence following lumpectomy, or accepting a mastectomy.

The advantages of a mastectomy are that no radiation therapy is required, and there is a decreased risk of local recurrence. Some women prefer the procedure because of the peace of mind they expect after the removal of the breast.

The disadvantages include more extensive surgery, and the emotional impact of losing the entire breast, including the nipple.

Your choice will be dictated by various factors. Here are a few considerations that would favor mastectomy over lumpectomy:

- The tumor is so big or the breast is so small that the cosmetic result would not be satisfactory after tumor removal.

- There is more than one tumor location in the breast.

- You are unwilling or unable to undergo radiation treatment.

- You prefer to have a mastectomy.

Remember that no decision needs to be made overnight. You can take up to several weeks to gather information. And you do not need to make the decision alone. Consult your healthcare professionals, consider getting a second opinion, and talk things over with your loved ones.

Patient advocacy organizations in your area can put you in touch with other women who had the same type of surgery that you are considering, and who will be happy to discuss your choice with you. See the Resources section for information on how to contact these organizations.

QUESTIONS TO ASK YOUR DOCTOR:

☐ Is lumpectomy an option for me? Why or why not?

☐ Does a mastectomy decrease the chances of the cancer coming back?

☐ How will I look after a mastectomy if I decide against reconstruction?

☐ Can you show me pictures?

☐ Can you refer me to a plastic surgeon so I can discuss my reconstruction options?

☐ What kind of reconstruction procedure do you think would be best for me?

☐ Who can I talk to about my concerns about appearance, dating, pregnancy, etc?

EXAMINING THE LYMPH NODES

Arteries and veins carry blood to and from various parts of the body. Some fluid seeps out of these blood vessels, and is returned to the blood stream by a network of thin tubes called lymphatic ducts. This fluid, called lymph, helps the body wash away foreign particles or other debris that can collect in the spaces between cells.

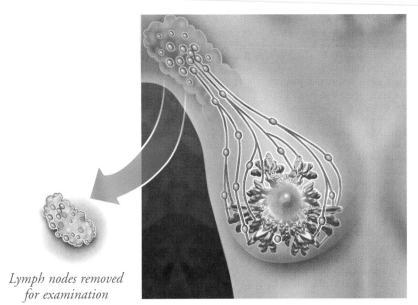

*Lymph nodes removed
for examination*

Lymphatic ducts from both the breast and the arm come together in the axilla, or armpit. There, the lymph is filtered through tiny bean-shaped organs called lymph nodes. Foreign particles (such as bacteria from an infection in the finger, or break-away cancer cells from a tumor in the breast) are trapped in the lymph nodes before they can enter the general circulation.

Whether you've had a mastectomy or a lumpectomy you may also have a procedure to remove some of the lymph nodes from your armpit and have them examined for evidence of cancer spread. Removing the lymph nodes does not help eliminate the cancer from your body. But determining whether cancer cells have spread to these lymph nodes is important for deciding what additional therapy will be needed.

AXILLARY LYMPH NODE DISSECTION

An axillary lymph node dissection can be done through a separate small incision in the armpit at the time of a lumpectomy, or through the main surgical incision as part of a mastectomy. The surgeon will remove a por-tion of the fat pad within which ten to twenty lymph nodes are imbedded. The tissue removed will be sent to the pathologist. Each node will be sliced and examined under the microscope for presence of cancer cells. The pathology report, which your physician will receive three to ten days after surgery, will indicate how many nodes were positive (in other words, had cancer cells in them).

An axillary lymph node dissection takes about an hour. The surgeon will need to exercise particular care to avoid injuring one of several important nerves that pass through this area.

Sentinel Lymph Node Biopsy

An important development in the staging of breast cancer is the increased use of a procedure called *sentinel lymph node biopsy* as an alternative to a full axillary node dissection. The principle is simple. As lymphatic fluid drains away from the breast, it first passes through certain lymph nodes located in key parts of the drainage system. These are called *sentinel nodes*, because they seem to act as gatekeepers. If the sentinel node is free of cancer, the odds are that there will be no cancer in the other nodes located downstream.

The procedure begins with the injection of a blue dye and/or of a small amount of radioactive material into the area near the tumor. The lymphatic fluid carries the dye to the first node in its path—the sentinel node. During surgery, the node is identified, removed and examined. If no cancer cells are found, a full dissection can be avoided.

This procedure takes longer, and requires a surgeon who is experienced in sentinel node biopsy, but it does help avoid the potentially serious complications such as damage to nerves and lymph ducts that can occur with the standard procedure.

After Axillary Lymph Node Dissection

After the surgery, a drain may be placed into the armpit to help remove blood and fluid that seeps out from the operated area.

Care for the incision is the same as for the lumpectomy or mastectomy: keeping it dry until the incision begins to heal and the drains are removed.

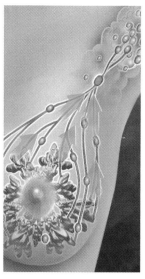

Lymphatic fluid drains toward the sentinel node

QUESTIONS TO ASK YOUR SURGEON

☐ Do you recommend that I have a sentinel lymph node biopsy instead of a full axillary lymph node dissection?

☐ What are the reasons for your recommendation?

☐ Are you and your surgical team experienced in performing this procedure?

Damage to one or more of the nerves that pass through the axilla, either accidentally or because the injury was unavoidable, may result in long term numbness in the armpit area, or weakness in some of the shoulder muscles. Often the numbness will improve over several years, but the sensitivity will never be normal. The weakness can generally be overcome with time.

Lymphedema

One of the more serious problems that may arise after an axillary lymph node dissection is a condition called lymphedema. It's caused by scarring of lymph vessels in the underarm area after removal of the lymph nodes and their connecting ducts. The circulation of lymph fluid is slowed, causing swelling of the arm, limiting its function, and making the arm more prone to infection.

As many as 10-20% of women undergoing axillary lymph node dissection will develop lymphedema of the arm. The condition may occur soon after surgery, or years later. While it is difficult to predict who will develop lymphedema, there are several precautions that you must take to help you avoid it. These include avoiding overusing the arm, and protecting it from skin infections and injuries.

For women who develop lymphedema, the treatment will focus on lymph-draining massage, special compression bandages, and special exercises, all under the supervision of a qualified therapist.

Arm swollen

Lymph drainage blocked by scarred ducts

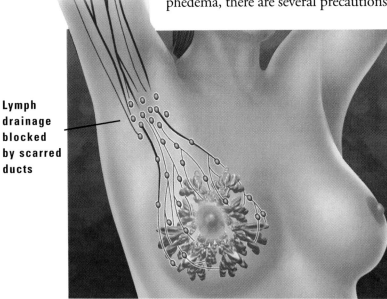

Lymphedema
swelling caused by blocked lymph ducts

Precautions that will help protect your arm from lymphedema

- Avoid sunburns or burns while cooking

- Have all injections, vaccinations, blood samples, and blood pressure tests done on the other arm whenever possible

- Use an electric razor with a narrow head for underarm shaving to reduce the risk of nicks or scratches

- Carry heavy packages or handbags on the other arm

- Wash cuts promptly, treat them with antibacterial medication, and cover them with a sterile bandage; check often for redness, soreness, or other signs of infection

- Never cut cuticles; use hand cream or lotion instead

- Wear watches or jewelry loosely, if at all, on the operated arm

- Wear protective gloves when gardening and when using strong detergents

- Use a thimble if you sew

- Avoid harsh chemicals and abrasive compounds

- Use insect repellent to avoid bites and stings

- Avoid tight elastic cuffs on blouses and nightgowns

- If your arm becomes red, swollen, or feels hot, call your doctor at once

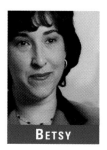

BETSY

I learned quickly that it was important to talk to doctors and nurses about not getting blood pressure taken or injections on the affected arm, to be careful when gardening, and what not. I do a lot of animal rescue and have to be careful with cat bites to the affected area.

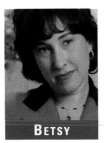

BETSY

The tumor was like a golf ball and it encompassed part of the nipple. The doctors explained that I would have to have the nipple removed and a large portion of the breast, even if I had a lumpectomy. My breasts aren't that large, so I opted for a mastectomy and breast reconstruction.

Here are some questions to consider when making your choice between mastectomy and lumpectomy:

- Is the appearance of my breast after surgery important to me?

- Is the sensitivity in my breast after surgery important to me?

- If I have breast-conserving surgery, am I willing to have a course of radiation therapy?

- If I have a mastectomy, do I also want breast reconstruction surgery?

- What treatment does my insurance cover, and what do I have to pay for?

CHAPTER 5

Reconstruction

After a mastectomy, the shape of the breast can be reconstructed using implants, or the patient's own tissues. It is important that you realize that reconstructive surgery cannot give you a new, normally functioning breast. It can only create a breast form which, under the best conditions, will have the shape and texture of your other breast.

For many women, a breast reconstruction after a mastectomy is a milestone that symbolizes that they have completed the treatment, and are ready to get on with their lives. It is also an opportunity to regain their feminine silhouette and restore their self-image.

Years ago, reconstructions were less common, partially because many cancers were discovered at an advanced stage, when long-term survival was not a certainty, and partially because reconstruction techniques left a lot to be desired.

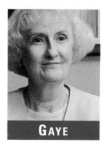

GAYE

I think when I had my surgery, I wasn't sure that I wanted reconstruction. It happened so fast that looking back, I think I probably would have asked for a consultation with a plastic surgeon.

Planning breast reconstruction

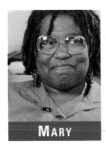

MARY

I went out to get my prosthesis. I went to a very small shop and I took a friend along with me who helped a lot. They have different color prostheses now. I was able to get one that worked for my skin tone. So that was really nice.

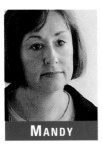

MANDY

After sixteen years, my silicone implants moved out of place. So I decided to have them replaced. I was back to work in about a week.

Today, almost any woman who has had a mastectomy can have her breast reconstructed. The new techniques yield excellent cosmetic results.

Myths about the disadvantages of reconstruction—such as presumed difficulty in detecting future recurrence—have been disproved. In addition, cost issues are also less of a factor, because coverage by insurance companies is now mandated by law.

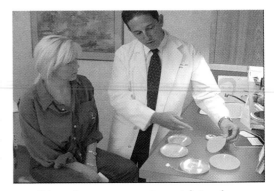

Discussing reconstruction with implants

RECONSTRUCTION TECHNIQUES

There are a number of techniques available to build a new breast mound, create a new nipple and areola, and make changes in the other breast to achieve better symmetry.

If you are considering reconstruction, even if it's to be done at a later date, arrange a meeting with a plastic surgeon well before your mastectomy, to discuss the details of the procedure. If your primary surgeon works closely with the plastic surgeon, the process will be smoother, and the results will be better.

Very commonly, you may need a minor plastic procedure on the other breast, such as a breast lift, to achieve the best similarity possible to the reconstructed breast.

Reconstruction may be easier if you have a skin-sparing mastectomy, where much of the skin of the breast is left in place. However, this procedure may carry an increased risk of local breast cancer recurrence. Discuss the safety of this option with both the breast surgeon and the plastic surgeon.

CHOOSING A PLASTIC SURGEON

For your reconstruction, it is crucial that you select a surgeon who has extensive experience in reconstructive breast surgery, and is a board-certified specialist, because the cosmetic results will depend significantly on the surgeon's skill. Your primary surgeon can refer you to one, or you can get a list of names in your area by contacting the American Society of Plastic Surgeons, listed in the Resources section.

One more key point: it is important that your expectations be realistic. The new breast can look natural, and feel normal to someone touching it, but you will not have sensation in the nipple, and will have decreased or no sensation in the skin of the breast. Your satisfaction with the final result will depend as much on the surgeon's skill and technique used, as on your healing pattern and your expectations.

RECONSTRUCTION OPTIONS

Reconstruction can be done at any time: at the time of mastectomy—which is called immediate reconstruction—or at a later date—which is called delayed reconstruction.

There are two main methods for reconstruction. One uses synthetic implants to create the shape of a breast. The other, the patient's own tissues, transplanted from another area of the body. Both methods are undergoing constant improvements and refinements.

Once the breast is rebuilt, you can go on to have a reconstruction of the nipple and the areola, to achieve an even more natural look. You may also benefit from cosmetic surgery on the other breast for better symmetry.

RECONSTRUCTION WITH SYNTHETIC IMPLANTS

The most common method of breast reconstruction is with implants. Synthetic implants are teardrop-shaped pouches that are inserted under the skin to create the form of a breast. The pouch is made of silicone, and is filled with saline (salt water solution) or with silicone gel.

In the early 1990's silicone was a source of concern because of a possible link to certain connective tissue diseases. Recent studies have shown that these suspicions were unfounded, and silicone implants continue to be available for breast reconstruction.

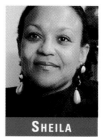

SHEILA

In the beginning, I started out with external prostheses. I didn't realize that I would end up with double D's again. These things are heavy! Wearing them eight hours gave me chest pain, backache, and headache, and so pretty soon, I began leaving them in the drawer, except when I needed to look "normal." And then I decided… "reconstruction."

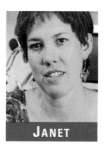

JANET

It didn't seem that important at first, but finally having a reconstruction did wonders for my confidence. Now when I look in the mirror, I don't cringe. When I change in the locker room, I don't hide. In my own mind, I'm a woman again.

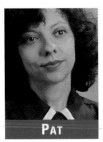

PAT

I had reconstruction at the time of the mastectomy. They put in an expander and slowly filled that for three months and then put in a permanent silicone implant. I am very happy with it.

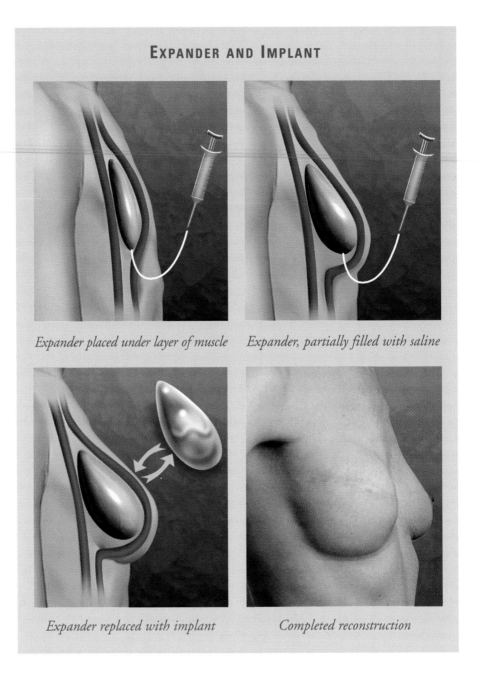

EXPANDER AND IMPLANT

Expander placed under layer of muscle   *Expander, partially filled with saline*

Expander replaced with implant   *Completed reconstruction*

You'll meet with a plastic surgeon before your mastectomy to choose an implant that will match your other breast and provide a pleasing, symmetrical appearance.

If you're having immediate reconstruction, the plastic surgeon will take over right after the mastectomy, while you're still under anesthesia. This part of the surgery will take about an hour.

In order to achieve the most pleasant shape and feel for the reconstructed breast, the implant is usually placed under the muscle, rather than directly under the skin.

If the implant is small, and sufficient skin from the breast remains in place, the surgeon may be able to insert the implant without undue stretch to the skin and muscles of your chest wall. Your reconstruction will be complete. However, if the implant is too large, the surgeon will need to use a temporary expander.

The expander is an elastic bag equipped with a fill tube and a valve. After the expander is inserted in place, it is filled with a small amount of saline. You'll return to the surgeon's office every week or two to have more saline injected into the expander. Gradually, over three to six months, the skin and muscle will stretch, just like they do over the abdomen during pregnancy. Then the expander will be removed and the permanent implant inserted in its place. A nipple and areola can be created during a future procedure.

A new type of implant, the Becker implant, has been recently re-introduced. It is a pouch that can first be used as an expander. Then, when the skin is sufficiently stretched, the fill tube is removed in a minor office procedure, and the pouch is left behind as a permanent implant. This is called a one-stage reconstruction, and can eliminate an extra surgical procedure.

After surgery

The first 24 to 72 hours after your initial implant surgery is when you experience the most discomfort. Your breast will be swollen and tender. Although every woman's recovery time is different, you should be able to resume many of your regular activities after about one week. You will need to wait at least one month before doing anything strenuous.

During the several weeks required to fully inflate the expander, you will probably have a feeling of fullness in your breast, but no major discomfort.

QUESTIONS TO ASK YOUR PLASTIC SURGEON:

☐ What type of reconstruction do you think is best for me?

☐ Will an implant make it more difficult to detect a local recurrence?

☐ What should I know about the "skin-sparing" mastectomy?

☐ What is the latest information regarding the safety of silicone implants?

☐ Can you show me pictures of reconstruction procedures you have done?

☐ Could I meet with some of the women so I can see and feel their breasts?

☐ Will my insurance pay for the reconstruction, even if it is done later? Will it pay for a breast prosthesis?

☐ Will I have a lot of pain? How can the pain be treated?

RECONSTRUCTION WITH YOUR OWN TISSUES

Breast reconstruction can be done using skin, muscle, and fat taken from another part of your body. This tissue transfer is called a myocutaneous flap, musculocutaneous flap, or simply, a flap.

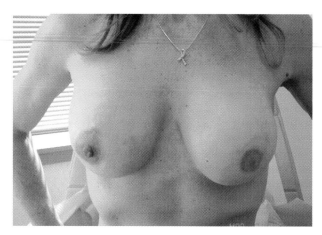

There are different types of myocutaneous flaps. Some, (like TRAM flaps and latissimus dorsi flaps), move tissues from an area of the body to the breast area, while preserving the original blood supply. Others, (like the DIEP, SIEP, or IGAP) are free flaps—the original blood supply to the transplanted tissue is cut then reconstructed.

Results of breast reconstruction (left breast)

TRAM (Transverse Rectus Abdominis) Flap

The TRAM flap has been one of the most common flaps for years. It uses one of the rectus abdominis muscles—the "abs," as weight lifters call them. The muscle, fat, and skin are separated from their natural attachments, and pulled up, under the skin, to the breast area. The flap is then shaped into the form of a breast. Some of the original blood supply is preserved.

The TRAM flap is the most versatile of the tissue flaps, and can usually create a good match to the other breast for all but the largest-breasted women. No implant is required as is often the case with the latissimus dorsi flap.

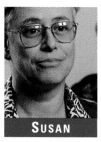

SUSAN

I had the buttock flap, and wound up with a tiny scar on my behind that you can hardly see, and a firm breast. And as soon as I was out of the hospital, I went straight to lunch with a friend.

The procedure takes three to five hours, and usually requires a four to seven day hospital stay. It also entails an abdominal incision, and does result in significant discomfort for some time after the surgery.

Rarely, a hernia may develop in the area from where the muscle was taken. But an additional cosmetic benefit of a TRAM flap is that it also gives the woman a "tummy tuck" as part of the procedure.

TRAM FLAP

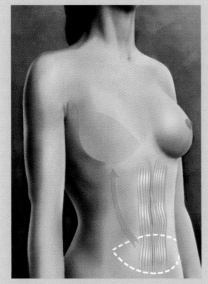

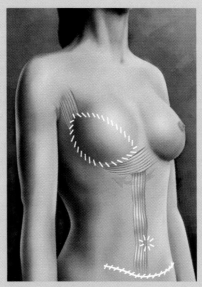

Tissue from the abdomen is used to create a breast mound

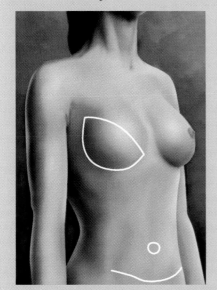

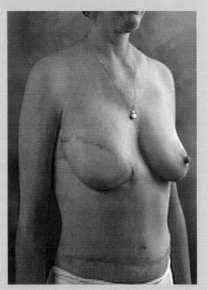

Completed reconstruction includes a "tummy tuck"

QUESTIONS TO ASK YOUR INSURANCE COMPANY:

☐ Does my policy cover the costs of the implant surgery, the implant anesthesia, and other related hospital costs? To what extent?

☐ Does it cover treatments for medical problems that may be caused by the implant or the reconstruction?

☐ Does it cover removal of the implants if this becomes necessary?

☐ If I choose to delay reconstruction and my company changes insurance plans, will I still be covered for breast reconstruction at a later date?

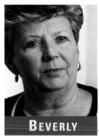

I went for the one with the perforating vessels. I had to stay in the hospital for four or five days. They watched the flap to make sure it was taking. But I was surprised that I was able to drive pretty much as soon as I got home. And the breast looks great!

Latissimus Dorsi Flap

The latissimus dorsi flap is sometimes referred to as Lat flap. For this procedure, an incision is made under the shoulder blade, and a temporary tunnel is created under the skin, just like for the TRAM flap. A portion of the latissimus dorsi muscle from the upper back, and the fat and skin covering it, are pulled through this tunnel and relocated to the breast area.

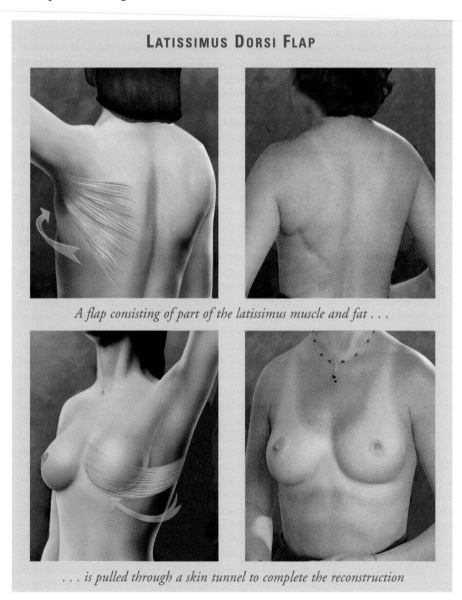

LATISSIMUS DORSI FLAP

A flap consisting of part of the latissimus muscle and fat . . .

. . . is pulled through a skin tunnel to complete the reconstruction

For most women, the latissimus muscle does not provide enough bulk to match the opposite breast, so a synthetic implant is added to make the reconstructed breast larger.

The procedure takes five to six hours and is done under general anesthesia.

Free Flap

To create a free flap, a portion of muscle, fat, and skin is removed from the abdomen or buttocks, and transplanted to the breast site. The original blood supply to the flap is cut, and then reconnected to a new artery and vein in the breast area. This procedure requires a plastic surgeon who is skilled in micro-surgery, because it involves sewing together blood vessels so thin, that the work must be done under a microscope.

Several more advanced forms of free flaps are gaining popularity. They use the so-called perforator vessels—blood vessels that branch off a deep artery and pass through the muscle, on the way to the fat and skin. The plastic surgeon isolates these vessels from the bigger artery, and dissects them out through the muscle, rather than taking them with the muscle. This technique offers the benefit of a longer blood vessel that is easier to re-attach in the breast area. By preserving the muscle, the patient's recovery is shorter, there is much less discomfort after surgery.

One example of a perforator flap is the DIEP (deep inferior epigastric perforator) flap. This flap uses fat and skin from the same area as the TRAM flap, but does not disturb the muscle. Recovery time is shorter, post-operative discomfort is less. In addition, the muscle in the donor area is not damaged, and retains its shape and function, unlike for the traditional TRAM flap, in which most, if not all the muscle is removed. A welcome by-product of the DIEP flap procedure is a tummy tuck.

Another option in free flaps is the IGAP flap that uses the inferior gluteal artery and a portion of the buttock tissue. The location of the donor site can be effectively concealed, and the outline of the buttock preserved.

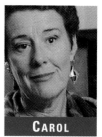

CAROL

One of the really good things about having reconstruction immediately, was that I woke up with a breast. Or something that passed for a breast, anyway. Now that it's healed, I can wear clothes that are tight or very low cut, and I don't have to worry about how I look.

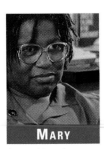

MARY

I considered reconstruction. But I'm not sure if I am going to have it. I have a lot of strong feelings about man-made products in my body and if I can't use the tissues from my own body, I don't think I will ever have it.

After Surgery

Your post-operative course will depend on the procedure you had, and on your body's ability to heal.

For some of the more complex free flap procedures, you will spend 24 hours in the intensive care unit, where you will have frequent checks to ensure that the blood supply to the flap is adequate. Then you will be transferred to a regular floor to continue your convalescence.

At home the care of the wound will be almost the same as if you only had a mastectomy. Generally, you will have additional drains in place, that will need to be drained by you or your care giver several times a day for the first few days. Most women can resume their activities of daily living within the week.

All flap reconstructions are complicated procedures and involve certain risks. Large portions of tissues are moved, and their blood supply is disrupted. There is a possibility that the flap will necrose, or die. This would require removal of the flap, causing significant discomfort and possible deformity.

Flaps cause pain both at the donor site and in the breast area. Removal of muscles from their original position can cause pain and weakness, or rarely, a hernia in the donor area.

On the other hand, the use of flaps avoids placing foreign materials into your body, and can result in the most natural-looking reconstructions. Many women—and their partners—appreciate the fact that the breast feels more natural than after an implant reconstruction.

Nipple and Areola Reconstruction

Women who want their reconstructed breast to look as natural as possible may choose to have a nipple and areola reconstruction. This procedure is usually done a few months after the breast reconstruction, so that the breast has had time to "settle" in place.

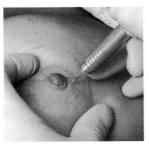

Areola is created by tattooing

Small flaps of skin on the reconstructed breast are raised and brought together into the shape of a nipple. The areola is created either from a skin graft, or by tattooing. The procedures can be done under local anesthesia.

WHICH IS RIGHT FOR ME?

Reconstruction is not for everyone, and it may not be right for you. Many women choose to do nothing, or to wear an artificial breast form.

If you decide to have breast reconstruction, your options will be many. Be sure to ask your plastic surgeon to show you photos, and perhaps arrange for you to interview some of the patients who had the same procedure. Here are some factors to keep in mind when making your decisions:

Synthetic Implants:

- They are not lifetime devices, and may rupture or need replacement.
- Implants may lead to capsular contracture, and misplacement.
- Some women report feeling the implant as a foreign object.
- Implants can be easily placed by most plastic surgeons.
- There is less surgery, less pain, shorter recovery, no additional scar, and less expense than with tissue flaps.

Tissue Flaps:

- They are typically soft and normal-appearing.
- There is no artificial implant in the body.
- With some flaps, a "tummy tuck" is an added bonus.
- There is lengthy, extensive, and expensive surgery, with blood transfusions and considerable post-operative discomfort.
- There is an additional scar at the donor site.
- There is a small but significant risk of the flap "not taking."

Immediate Reconstruction:

- You don't have to wake up from mastectomy surgery without a breast.
- One surgery rather than two means lower cost, fewer problems from anesthetic and surgery, and less recovery time.

Delayed Reconstruction:

- Provides additional time to make reconstructive choices.
- For the woman undergoing chemotherapy, possibly decreases the chance of infection in the reconstruction area.
- Avoids difficulties coordinating operative schedules, which may delay surgery.

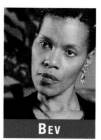

BEV

My surgeon didn't believe in immediate reconstruction. He didn't think the decision should be made at that time. As a matter of fact, he and my plastic surgeon had a disagreement about that, because my plastic surgeon believed that you should do it all together.

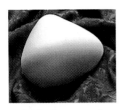

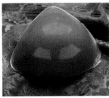

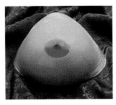

Prostheses are available in light-weight foam, or in natural-weight and silicone

EXTERNAL BREAST FORMS

Many women choose to have no reconstruction of any type after the mastectomy. Some make this decision because they want to avoid extra surgery. Others because they're comfortable with their appearance and body image. A few view their scars as battle scars from a war they waged. And yet others do want reconstruction to erase the visual reminder of cancer, or to enhance their self-image. There is no right or wrong answer, and your decision must be respected by those who are close to you, and by your healthcare team.

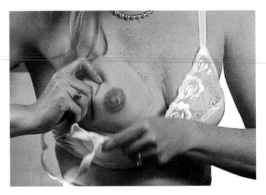

Lifelike prostheses can be custom-made

If you choose to have no reconstruction, you may want to use a breast form instead. Breast forms, or prostheses as they are also called, are available in a variety of sizes, shapes, and colors. Some are designed to fit into a special bra. Others can be attached securely to your chest using a special adhesive. Prostheses range from inexpensive foam inserts to custom-molded replacements with realistic color and texture, designed to duplicate your natural breast as exactly as possible.

Breast forms are used not just to maintain appearance and sense of balance. They play an important functional role by relieving the uneven strain on your posture that may occur after a mastectomy, particularly if your breasts are large.

The decision to have reconstruction or to wear an external prosthesis is a very personal one, and is based on your feelings about your body, your sexuality, and your tolerance for additional surgery. Your decision is legitimate, and must be respected by your healthcare providers and your loved ones.

CHAPTER 6

Radiation Therapy

Radiation therapy is a form of treatment that uses the same type of rays—commonly called X-rays—that are used to create an image of the chest, or of a broken bone. For treatment purposes, the X-rays are of higher intensity. High doses of radiation can destroy the ability of cells to grow and multiply. Both normal and cancer cells are affected, but normal cells can recover quickly, while the abnormal, rapidly multiplying cancer cells, are permanently damaged. Giving a course of radiation therapy after a lumpectomy can help ensure that no cancer cells remain in the breast area.

Unlike chemotherapy—a systemic treatment that treats the entire body—radiation therapy is considered a local treatment, because it treats only the cancer area.

Radiation therapy is administered at medical centers staffed by teams of professionals specializing in radiation oncology. There are two ways to administer radiation therapy. The oldest and most common, external beam radiation therapy, or EBRT, uses a complex device that aims the beam at the breast area from several angles. A newer method is brachytherapy. It relies on tiny radioactive seeds placed temporarily directly into the breast.

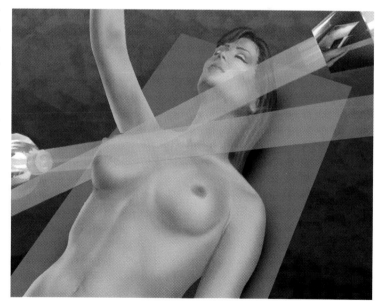

Radiation beams are directed from several angles.

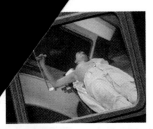

The staff will monitor you at all times.

EXTERNAL BEAM RADIATION THERAPY

Treatment Planning

A full course of external beam radiation therapy spans five to seven weeks. The goal is to deliver the optimal dose to the breast area, with the least impact on the surrounding normal tissues. This requires an approach carefully tailored to each case.

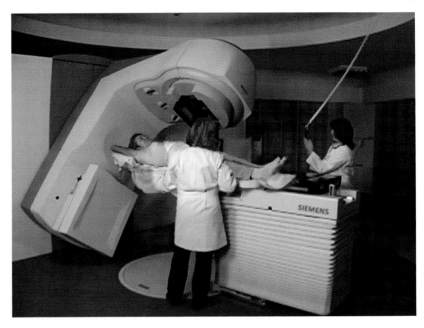

External Beam Radiation Therapy is delivered by a linear accelerator

Using a simulation unit, the radiation oncologist staff will determine the best angles for the beam. Then they will outline the treatment ports—places on your body where the beam will be aimed. These ports will be temporarily marked with colored ink. Don't wash these marks off until you're told to do so. Later, they may be replaced by tiny tattoos. These markings will ensure that the beam is aimed accurately every treatment session.

The simulation may take several hours. The information obtained will be entered into a computer to develop your treatment plan. Sometimes a special cast will be fabricated for your chest to ensure consistent positioning. Once the planning is completed, the treatments can begin.

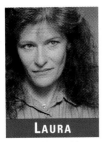

LAURA

The staff would meet me promptly, and take me right in, set me up, and make sure that I was comfortable. The session always went by really quickly, which was great. And they were very kind, very nice people, which made me less nervous.

How Treatment is Given

The first treatment will take longer than the others, in order to make sure the position matches the angles that were worked out during simulation.

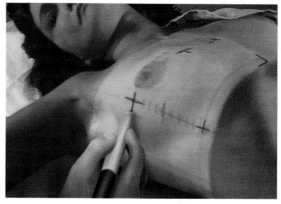

The treatments are given by a radiation therapist in accordance with the plan developed for you by the team. Typically, you will arrive at the facility at the appointed time each day. You may want to bring a friend for moral support during the first session or two. You may also want to bring an iPod or a book to read in case you have to wait.

The technologist marks the treatment ports

Don't use deodorant, because deodorants contain aluminum that may interfere with the radiation beam. Use cornstarch, or a prescription deodorant recommended by your physician. Wear a two-piece outfit so you can change easily into a patient gown from the waist up.

The treatment is given in a room that has thick concrete walls and lead-lined doors, to protect those who are outside the treatment area from radiation. The device used to deliver radiation is called a linear accelerator. At first the whole set up may seem complex and intimidating. But don't be alarmed. A TV monitor lets the staff keep you in sight at all times, in case you need anything.

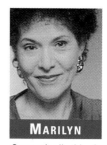

MARILYN

Cosmetically, I had very good results from the treatment. If you look at my breasts right now, you couldn't tell that there was treatment done to one breast as opposed to the other breast. They look exactly the same.

The radiation therapist will adjust the position of the machine according to the previously determined settings, then step out of the room. During the actual exposure you must remain as still as possible. The unit will be repositioned one or two times to change the angle of the beam. Each exposure lasts only a few minutes and you won't see or feel anything.

The full course of treatment runs about five weeks, with sessions from Monday through Friday, and rest and recovery periods during weekends. If you have to miss a day or two, discuss the situation with your doctor or nurse. You can make up the days at the end, but the efficiency of the treatment depends on having as few delays as possible.

QUESTIONS TO ASK
YOUR DOCTOR:

☐ Why do I need radiation
  therapy?

☐ How is the radiation
  oncologist (physician)
  involved if the treat-
  ments are given by the
  therapists?

☐ How will I evaluate the
  effectiveness of the
  treatments?

☐ Which method is better
  for me, external beam
  or brachytherapy?

☐ Can I continue my usual
  work or exercise
  schedule?

☐ Can I miss a few treat-
  ments?

☐ Can I arrange to be
  treated elsewhere if I
  am traveling?

☐ What side effects, if
  they occur, should I
  report immediately?

☐ Can I expose the treat-
  ed area to the sun?

☐ Will I be able to con-
  ceive and bear a child
  after treatments?

☐ What about the differ-
  ent cost of brachytherapy vs. external beam?

The start of your therapy will depend on whether you are also undergoing chemotherapy. Depending on the practices of the facility where you are being treated, you may have chemotherapy and radiotherapy simultaneously, or be started on chemotherapy, then treated with radiation, then again with chemotherapy. Sometimes the delay may be as long as several weeks or several months. There is little danger of the cancer cells spreading during this delay.

SIDE EFFECTS OF EXTERNAL BEAM RADIATION THERAPY

Radiation therapy is a safe, proven treatment with few unwanted side effects. Most of them are not serious and disappear quickly. The most common are fatigue and skin changes. You will not have nausea or lose your hair, as you might with chemotherapy, and you certainly won't be radioactive. Most people find that they can go through radiation therapy while maintaining their normal work schedule and lifestyle.

Caring for Your Skin During Radiation Therapy

- Be extra kind to skin in the treatment area. Don't use any soaps, lotions, deodorants, cosmetics, talcum powder, or other substances in the treated area without talking with your doctor.

- Do not use adhesive tape on treated skin. If bandaging is necessary, use paper tape. Apply the tape outside of the treatment area.

- Do not apply heating pads or ice packs to the area. Use only lukewarm water for bathing the treated area.

- Use an electric shaver if you must shave the area—but only after checking with your doctor or nurse.

- Protect the area from the sun. Cover the treated skin with light clothing before going outside. Ask your doctor if you should use a lotion that contains a sunblock. If so, use a PABA product with a protection factor of at least 15. Continue to protect your skin from sunlight for at least one year after radiation therapy.

Fatigue

Stress related to your illness, daily trips for treatment, and the effects of radiation on normal cells may lead to fatigue. Most people begin to feel tired after a few weeks of radiation therapy. You can help yourself by not trying to do too much. If you feel tired, limit your activities, use your leisure time in a restful way, and try to get more sleep at night.

If you continue working a full-time job while undergoing radiation therapy, talk with your employer about adjusting your work schedule, or try working at home for a period of time.

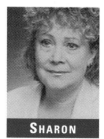

SHARON

The change in the breast that I noticed is that one's a little firmer. I nursed three babies so the breasts were eh-eh to begin with. I don't notice any other change. I don't care. As long it's over with and gone and all's healed and fine.

Skin Changes

The energy waves used in radiation therapy have an effect on the skin that resembles the effect of intense sunlight. Some skin irritation and redness, similar to a sunburn, may develop by the third or fourth week of treatment. Don't rub or scratch the affected area. Use mild soap, being careful not to wash off port markings, if you have any. Wear soft clothing, preferably cotton, and protect the treated area from sunlight. Advise your doctor or nurse at once if your skin cracks or blisters, so that they can instruct you on proper care.

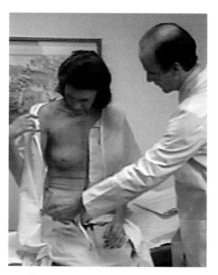

Skin redness caused by radiation

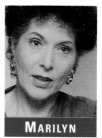

MARILYN

Toward the end of the treatment, I did experience some changes in the breast. I had been forewarned this would happen. There were some skin changes, some coloring changes, some tenderness. But, I had very little trouble really, compared to what might have happened.

Other Side Effects

Radiation therapy may cause breast swelling and tenderness, so you may find sleeping on your stomach uncomfortable. Try using pillows to create a comfortable position. The swelling will subside after treatment.

In addition, you may have tenderness in the breast and chest area for up to a year, but seldom will it be severe enough to require pain medication.

On a long term basis, the breast may become slightly smaller or larger. The breast may also become slightly firmer, but significant hardening is rare.

BRACHYTHERAPY

Another method for treating the breast area is brachytherapy. Instead of an external beam, brachytherapy uses a radioactive source that is placed directly into the area where the tumor was. There are two brachytherapy methods: interstitial and single-balloon.

For interstitial brachytherapy, 10-20 thin, hollow plastic tubes will be inserted into the breast. A machine called an Afterloader will thread the radioactive source into each hollow tube, one at a time. A CT scan and a computerized program plot the precise placement of radioactive source to insure that the entire area receives an even dose of radiation. After the treatment, which last 5-10 minutes, you will be free to go home. You will have a total of ten treatments over five days.

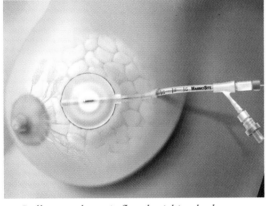

Single-catheter brachytherapy works on a similar principle. After the cancerous lump is removed, the surgeon places a thin tube with a balloon at the end, into the breast, and inflates the balloon with saline, creating a space.

For the treatment itself, a small radioactive pellet is threaded through the tube into the balloon, and left in place for five minutes. This procedure is repeated twice a day for five days. You are free to leave the hospital between treatments.

Balloon catheter inflated within the breast

Studies have shown that brachytherapy and external beam therapy are similarly effective in destroying cancer cells within the breast, and reducing the chance of local cancer recurrence.

Brachytherapy creates a higher intensity nearest the tumor site, with less spillover to surrounding normal tissues, such as lungs or heart.

The main advantage of brachytherapy is that women who do not have easy access to a radiation therapy facility five days a week, for five to seven weeks, can complete a course of treatment in five days. This may make the difference between choosing lumpectomy with radiation, or settling for a mastectomy.

CHAPTER 7

Chemotherapy

Local treatments—surgery and radiation therapy—treat cancer cells in the breast area only. But if there is reason to suspect that cancer cells have traveled outside the breast area, you will need a systemic treatment, using drugs that can reach all parts of the body. This treatment can be in the form of chemotherapy (drugs that kill cancer cells), hormonal therapy (drugs that prevent cancer cells from growing), immunotherapy (drugs that help your body fight off cancer), or a combination of these.

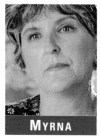

MYRNA

What I associated with chemo was sickness, nausea, not being able to function in my life. The reality has been amazing. I never expected to do as well as I did. I have virtually no problems whatsoever. I've been able to go about my life completely normally.

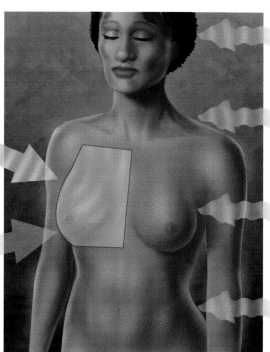

LOCAL TREATMENTS

SYSTEMIC TREATMENTS

Radiation Therapy

Chemotherapy

Surgery

Hormonal Therapy

Immunomotherapy

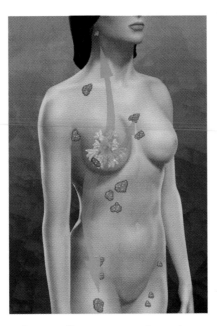

Cancer cells can metastasize to lung, bone, liver, and other organs

Why would you need additional therapy if there are no signs of tumor spread to other areas?

The problem with cancer is that as the tumor grows, cancer cells can break away and travel down blood vessels or lymph ducts to other parts of the body—much the same way as seeds from a weed are carried away by the wind, or float down a river, to grow somewhere else.

In the very early stages, these groups of break-away cells, called micrometastases, are very small, and cannot be found by any test or method that exists today. But if one waits until they grow into larger tumors, called metastases, that can be confirmed by X-rays or CT scans, then successful treatment becomes difficult.

So if there is any reason to suspect that cells from your tumor had a chance to metastasize to other parts of your body before the cancer was removed, you may be treated with chemotherapy or hormonal therapy to destroy those tumor cells as soon as possible.

WHAT IS CHEMOTHERAPY?

Chemotherapy uses drugs, called cytotoxic (cell-killing) drugs, to destroy cancer cells. It is often used as additional, or adjuvant therapy, in conjunction with local treatments like surgery and radiation therapy.

Chemotherapy can also be given before surgery to shrink a tumor. This pretreatment is called neo-adjuvant chemotherapy. Chemotherapy may also be used for treating metastatic disease—tumors that have spread to other parts of the body.

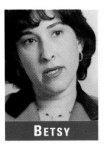

BETSY

I was actually far more fearful and anxious about chemotherapy than I was about losing my breast. And to a large degree that fear and anxiety were unfounded, because the chemo wasn't that bad.

When first told that they have breast cancer, many women panic at the thought of having to go through chemotherapy, because they have heard of chemotherapy as something that makes you deathly ill, or makes your hair fall out. "Will I have to have chemo?" is one of the first questions that many women ask.

Much has changed in recent years. Today there are very effective drugs that can greatly reduce—and sometimes eliminate—the side effects of chemotherapy, making the experience much more tolerable than it was rumored to be in the past.

Do you personally need chemotherapy? This decision will not be made until after the initial surgery. At that time, your team of physicians will review all the data, including tumor size and spread to lymph nodes, and calculate your risk of having micrometastases.

The question of whether to use chemotherapy is a complex issue, and you need to participate in the decision process.

Here is one way for you to evaluate the possible benefits: Chemotherapy reduces the risk of recurrence by about one third. So if the risk that your cancer has spread is high—say, 60%—chemotherapy will improve your odds by a third (20%). In other words, your risk of recurrence will go down from 60% to 40%. That's a significant improvement.

But suppose your cancer is not very aggressive, or the tumor was small, and your physician estimates that your chance of a recurrence is only 6%. Now a reduction by a third amounts to only 2%—from 6% down to 4%. That is a very small improvement, and may not be worth the side effects that you may have.

Your physicians will help you evaluate objectively the expected advantages and disadvantages of chemotherapy. And remember, if you decide on chemotherapy, you will enjoy the benefits of one of the most powerful tools for fighting breast cancer available today.

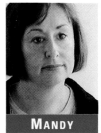

MANDY

I had a severe reaction and became so weak that I couldn't get out of bed for a day. Finally, I crawled on my hands and knees to the bathroom, and took a shower sitting on the floor. A few days later I awakened with an euphoric feeling. I knew I would be cured. The worst had passed and the rest would be a downhill ride. All I needed to do was hang on.

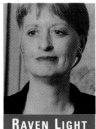

RAVEN LIGHT

I am not a suicidal person. I love life. The first set of chemotherapy that I did was on a Friday afternoon, and that night I vomited all night long. The next day, I just thought of ways to kill myself. I had no libido. I had no interest in sex. I had hardly any energy. It was the pits.

**QUESTIONS TO ASK
YOUR DOCTOR:**

☐ Do I need chemo-
therapy? Why?

☐ What drugs do you
recommend?

☐ What are the benefits
and risks of chemo-
therapy?

☐ How successful is this
treatment for the type of
cancer I have?

☐ How will you evaluate
the effectiveness of the
treatments?

☐ What side effects will I
experience?

☐ Can I work while I'm
having chemotherapy?

☐ Can I travel between
treatments (short busi-
ness or pleasure trips)?

☐ What other limitations
can I expect?

HOW CHEMOTHERAPY WORKS

Cells go through several steps in the process of cell division. First, the genetic material (DNA) in the nucleus forms strands called chromosomes (see
step #1 in the diagram below). Then the chromosomes divide into two sets
(see step #2) and the body of the cell enlarges. Finally the cell splits into two
identical cells, each with its own set of DNA (step #3.) Chemotherapy drugs
interfere with various parts of this cycle, making it difficult for the cells to
reproduce and repair themselves.

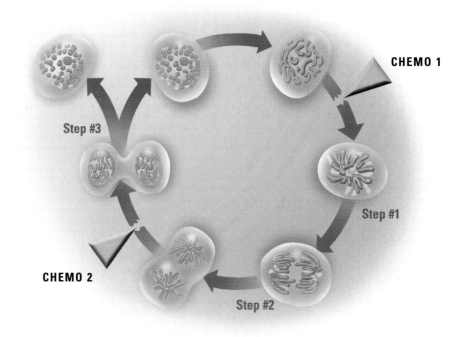

Different chemotherapy drugs affect different parts of the cell division cycle

Chemotherapy treatment affects both normal cells and cancer cells, but
because cancer cells generally divide more rapidly, and are less effective at
self-repair, they are more affected by the therapy than normal cells. As a
result, more cancer cells than normal cells are killed. With proper choice
and timing of chemotherapy, the tumor can be destroyed without excessive
damage to normal tissues.

There are dozens of different chemotherapy drugs, each designed to interfere with a different part of the cell's duplication process. By using a com-

bination of two or three different drugs, it is possible to affect several phases of the duplication cycle and increase the effectiveness of the treatment.

Your oncologist will recommend the best drug or combination of drugs, based on the characteristics of your tumor, degree of suspected spread, and your general health. You may want to participate actively in this decision. Some drug combinations are more likely than others to put you into early menopause, or make you sterile.

The most common drugs used for breast cancer are cyclophosphamide, methotrexate, fluorouracil (5-FU), Adriamycin and the taxane drugs Taxol and Taxotere.

Drugs are often given in combination. For example, CMF—which stands for cyclophosphamide, methotrexate, and fluorouracil; AC—for Adriamycin, and cyclophosphamide; TAC—Taxotere, Adriamycin and Cytoxan; or XT—Xeloda and Taxotere. Your physician will give you the latest information on new drug developments.

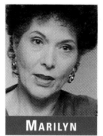

MARILYN

I actually did some modeling during the time I was on chemotherapy, which is sort of a contradiction in terms for many people. But, it really got me through what might have been a difficult period and it made it a very positive year for me.

HOW CHEMOTHERAPY IS GIVEN

Most chemotherapy drugs are given by injection into a vein, or IV. These injections can be given in a private doctor's office, in a hospital, or in a cancer center. Some chemotherapy drugs are given orally, and you take them just as you would any other pill. Taking the drugs orally requires more attention to timing and dosing on the part of the patient.

Chemotherapy is given in cycles. The cycle may be as short as one week, or as long as four weeks. This allows the normal cells in your body to recover between treatments. The full course of therapy takes three to six months.

Dose Dense Chemotherapy

In a new method called dose dense chemotherapy, drugs are given more frequently. Recent studies have shown that by keeping the doses the same, but reducing the interval between doses, it is possible to improve the outcome of the treatment in women whose cancers have spread to lymph nodes.

The decreased interval between doses may cause a decrease in red blood cell

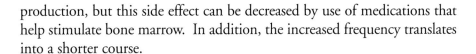

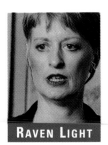

RAVEN LIGHT

One day my roommate came home with the flu, and I caught it. My white blood cell count was so low, I had to go to the hospital.

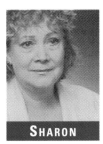

SHARON

The side effects that I had with chemo in the beginning were minimal. They increased. I gained a considerable amount of weight. I don't know if that was totally the chemo, or that I was saying, "Ahh, phooey. I'm going to eat whatever I want to eat." And part of me said I should be eating healthy, which I tried to do, but the other part of me said enjoy the ice cream bar too.

production, but this side effect can be decreased by use of medications that help stimulate bone marrow. In addition, the increased frequency translates into a shorter course.

Scientists are continuing to conduct studies to verify whether this very promising approach is equally effective in early stage cancers that have not yet spread.

Do not confuse "dose dense chemotherapy" with "bone marrow transplants" or "peripheral or stem cell harvesting." A few years ago clinicians attempted treating advanced breast cancer with extra-high doses of chemotherapy. To deal with the life-threatening damage to the bone marrow, the patient also underwent a procedure known as bone marrow transplant—her bone marrow cells where harvested, preserved by freezing, then reimplanted after chemotherapy. The procedure was complex and expensive. Unfortunately, recently completed studies showed that this procedure has no advantages over conventional treatment.

Typical IV Chemotherapy Day

Your experience with chemotherapy will vary depending on where you receive your treatments, but healthcare professionals realize that chemotherapy may be a stressful experience for you, and try to make your visit as pleasant as possible.

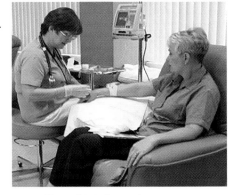

Typical IV chemotherapy room

You may make friends with some of the other patients who come for treatment at the same time. Bring a book or a portable music player, or practice relaxation or visualization, to make the session more pleasant. Depending on how you feel after treatments, you may want to ask a friend to come with you—for moral support, or to drive you home.

Before you receive the scheduled dose of chemotherapy, the nurse will draw your blood, to check whether the blood-producing cells in your bone marrow have adequately recovered, and to verify whether chemotherapy is affecting your liver or other organs. If the results of the tests are outside of normal limits, your oncologist may decide to lower the dose of chemo, or postpone the treatment.

If your results are acceptable, the nurse will take you to the treatment area and start the IV (intravenous line) through which the drug will be injected. If your veins are easy to reach, this will take a few seconds, and feel like a pinprick. Then the drug will be administered. Some drugs are given as a rapid injection, others are dripped in slowly over a longer period—sometimes up to three hours. Generally you won't feel any discomfort.

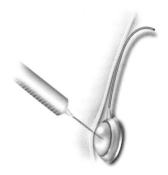

Chemotherapy drugs injected through a port

Vascular Access Devices

Sometimes veins are thin, damaged, or covered by a layer of fat, making it difficult for the nurse to start an IV line. In addition, a few chemo drugs can be very irritating to the veins, and over the course of treatment, can damage the vein at the injection site. In such cases a port may be installed under the skin.

Ports consist of a tube (catheter), attached to a dome-shaped part. The device is surgically implanted under the skin, with the dome placed in the chest or arm, where it will be easily accessible for injections through a needle. The catheter is threaded into a large vein, where rapid blood flow will dilute the drug, and keep it from damaging the lining of the vein. The whole device will be completely covered by skin, so it will not interfere with your activities. You can swim, bathe and exercise freely.

Ports can also be used for drawing blood, thus avoiding needle sticks of the arms during clinic visits.

SIDE EFFECTS OF CHEMOTHERAPY

Anti-cancer drugs work by preventing cells from growing and dividing. The effect is strongest on rapidly dividing cells such as cancer cells, but normal tissues can also be affected, particularly the gastrointestinal or GI tract, the bone marrow, hair follicles and the reproductive system. So the most common side effects are related to these organs, and include nausea, fatigue, menopausal symptoms and hair loss. The side effects will vary with the drug used, and with your own tolerance to it.

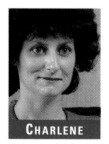

CHARLENE

My physician had given me several different anti-emetics to find the absolute best for me to combat the nausea and vomiting. I will say that it definitely was trial and error. Some did not work for me, others helped a lot.

**QUESTIONS TO ASK
YOUR DOCTOR:**

☐ How can I manage
nausea?

☐ Will I be given medica-
tions to treat side
effects?

☐ Can I take public
transportation home
after treatments?

☐ Should I eat before
I come for my
treatments?

☐ Can I take vitamins or
herbs if I choose?

While it is important to be prepared for possible side effects of chemotherapy, it is equally important not to assume that you will have all, many, or even a few of them. Many people go through chemotherapy without significant ill effects.

Don't compare your treatment with that of another patient, because there are so many different varieties of breast cancer, and so many variables on which the decision is based. Also, do not be alarmed by other women's reports about side effects. Their drugs, and their ability to tolerate them, may be quite different from yours. And remember, if you don't have side effects, it does not mean that the drugs are not working.

It's not likely that you will ever look forward to your chemotherapy days, but a positive attitude, help from your healthcare team, and support from your friends and family can make chemotherapy a tolerable experience.

Nausea

Today, thanks to powerful antiemetic drugs, such as Kytril and others, nausea is much less common than in years past. There are several effective medications available that will control, if not completely eliminate, nausea. Discuss this with your healthcare professionals, and make sure that you are receiving the best anti-nausea medication for your particular needs.

In addition to medications, consider other options, such as relaxation or imagery, that have proven to be quite effective for many patients. You can find more information on this subject in Chapter 9.

Nausea can lead to loss of appetite. Since good nutrition is very important to help you fight cancer and retain strength, you should make sure that you have adequate food intake, especially proteins and fluids. Eat small frequent meals avoiding stomach-bloating carbonated liquids.

If you do experience nausea, it usually won't be until for hours or even days after the injection. It may last from a few hours to up to several days, depending on the individual person. In rare instances, the nausea can be severe. Sometimes even the fear of nausea itself is so bad that a woman becomes nauseated at the mere sight of the medication, or of the nurse administering it. This is called *anticipatory nausea*.

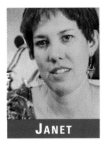

JANET

The first cycle, I didn't really have any side effects. The second one brought cramping and diarrhea, watery eyes, dry mouth, sores in my mouth. With each cycle, the side effects increased. After about three or four, my onco-logist cut back the chemicals.

A few simple steps that can relieve nausea:

- Remove dentures on days you receive drug treatments.

- Try breathing through your mouth when you feel nauseated.

- Avoid fried or other fatty foods.

- Hold a mint or lemon drop in your mouth.

- Avoid eating your favorite foods when you are nauseated, so that you do not develop an aversion to them.

- If the smell of food makes you nauseated, cook outside or take a walk while the food is being prepared.

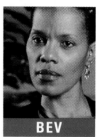

BEV

I would go to the gym and from the gym to get my chemo, then leave chemo and go running. From what I learned, it was just a matter of adjusting my anti-nausea meds.

Remember, effective control of nausea may make the difference between completing the full course of therapy, or quitting too early.

Despite the possible loss of appetite, many women notice an increase in weight as a result of treatment with most chemotherapy drugs. Weight gain of up to twenty pounds is not uncommon, and can be a distressing side effect. For the sake of maintaining your well being, be cautious of any weight gain.

Fatigue

Chemotherapy can make you feel tired, especially on the first day after each treatment. Adjust your schedule so that you can rest if you want.

Many women find that given some flexibility they can keep a fairly normal level of activity. If you feel totally unable to function at a reasonable level, tell your oncologist about it. Your drug dose may be too high, and may need to be readjusted. In addition, your physician may recommend medications to help your body rebuild red blood cells, which may increase your energy level.

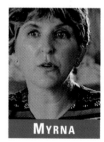

MYRNA

I had contacted my beautician and got two wigs before the hair came out. So the first day, as soon as it started flying, I had the wigs on and they've been fine.

Hair Loss

One of the side effects of chemotherapy that causes women the most sadness is hair loss. How much hair you lose—some or all—will depend on which drugs you are getting. The good news is that hair lost due to chemotherapy always grows back, sometimes thicker than it was originally.

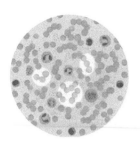

Red blood cells

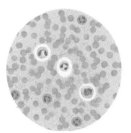

White blood cells

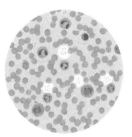

Platelets

Usually hair falls out over a period of a few weeks, starting around the third week after the first dose of chemotherapy. You may find large clumps on your pillow, or in the shower, or notice a lot of hair in your comb. Some women experience a sudden loss of hair.

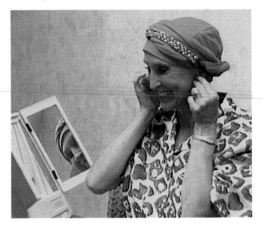

Buy a wig before your hair falls out, and try to pick one that resembles your natural hair. Insurance may cover some of the cost. Ask your beautician to style your wig the way you usually wear your hair.

Look Good...Feel Better is a public service program sponsored by the Cosmetic, Toiletry, and Fragrance Association Foundation in partnership with the American Cancer Society and the National Cosmetology Association. The program helps women manage changes in their appearance resulting from cancer treatment. You will find their contact information in the Resources section.

Bone Marrow Suppression

Bone marrow cells, which produce red blood cells, white blood cells, and platelets in your blood, are particularly affected by chemotherapy, and may lose some, or all, of their function, leading to lower blood cell counts.

Red blood cells (RBC's) transport oxygen. The normal value, measured in mg (milligrams) of hemoglobin (Hb, the oxygen carrying protein in the cell) is twelve to fourteen. A low red blood cell count, called anemia, will generally give you fatigue.

White blood cells (WBC's) help fight infection. A normal WBC count is in the 4,000-10,000 range. There are several different types of white blood cells. The most important for fighting infection are called neutrophils. Oncologists use the absolute neutrophil count (ANC) to monitor patients under treatment, and to determine whether the next dose can be given. A neutrophil count of less than 1000 is called neutropenia, and makes you susceptible to colds or infections, including skin wound infections.

Platelets help the blood clot. A low platelet count, below 150,000, can predispose to bleeding. This can take the form of excessive bleeding from wounds, or slow bleeding into the stomach or intestine, which could appear as black stools.

Your chemotherapy dose will be adjusted to achieve the maximum effect on the tumor cells, without dangerously impairing the ability of the bone marrow to produce blood cells in sufficient quantities.

If your bone marrow becomes excessively suppressed, your doctor may add other medications to your treatment, to stimulate your bone marrow to produce more blood cells. Raising your white cell count will help you fight off infections. Raising your red cell count will give your blood more capacity to carry oxygen, and will improve your strength.

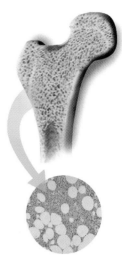

Microscopic view of bone marrow

Infections

When your white blood cell count is low, your body may not be able to fight off infections, even if you take extra care. Most infections come from bacteria normally found on the skin, in the intestines, and in the genital tract.

Be alert to signs that you might have an infection, such as:

- Fever over 100 degrees Fahrenheit
- Sweating and chills
- Loose bowels
- A burning feeling when you urinate
- A severe cough or sore throat
- Unusual vaginal discharge or itching
- Redness, swelling, or tenderness around a wound.

Report any signs of infection to your doctor right away. This is especially important when your white blood cell count is low. If you have a fever, don't use aspirin, acetaminophen (Tylenol), or any other medicine to bring your temperature down without first checking with your doctor.

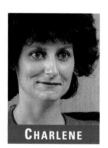

CHARLENE

The absolute very worst side effect, I still say to this day, has been the hair loss. That did me in. That was horrifying. When I was in the shower, all of a sudden it would just come out in my hand, crops of it. Emotionally it was a terrible roller coaster. Once it was gone, I felt more relieved. Then it was time to take the next step and move on.

**QUESTIONS TO ASK
YOUR DOCTOR:**

☐ Will I continue to have
my menstrual periods?

☐ If not, when will they
return?

☐ Should I use birth
control? What type do
you recommend?

☐ Will I be able to con-
ceive and bear a child
after treatments?

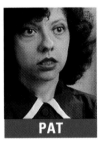

PAT

*While I was on chemotherapy,
I felt that I was actually doing
something to take charge of
the cancer, to kill any cancer
cells that might be running
amuck in my body. When I
walked out of the chemo suite
for the last time, there was a
feeling of "Now what? Where
do I go from here?"*

*When your white count is lower than normal, it is very important to try to
prevent infections by taking the following steps:*

• Wash your hands often. Be sure to wash them extra well before you
eat and before and after you use the bathroom.

• Clean your rectal area thoroughly after each bowel movement. Ask
your doctor or nurse for advice if the area becomes irritated. Check
with your doctor before using enemas or suppositories.

• Stay away from people who have diseases you can catch, such as a
cold, the flu, measles, or chickenpox. Try to avoid crowds.

• Stay away from children who recently have received
immunizations, such as vaccines for polio, measles or mumps.

• Don't cut or tear the cuticles off your nails.

• Be careful not to nick yourself when using sharp tools.

• Use an electric shaver instead of a razor to prevent cuts.

• Use a soft toothbrush that won't hurt your gums.

• Don't squeeze or scratch pimples.

• Take a warm (not hot) bath, shower, or sponge bath every day.
Pat your skin dry using a light touch. Don't rub.

• Use lotion or oil to soften and heal your skin if it becomes dry
and cracked.

• Clean cuts and scrapes right away with water and an antiseptic.

• Wear protective gloves when gardening or cleaning up after
animals and others, especially small children.

• Do not get any immunization shots without checking with your
doctor first.

NOTES ON ORAL CHEMOTHERAPY

If you are taking an oral chemotherapy drug, you need to be especially watchfull about side effects since you will be taking the medication at home away from the watchful eye of your healthcare providers. If you fail to inform your physician promptly about any side effects that you might be having, the side effects may become worse to the point that you may not be able to take the drug at all.

Be sure to find out what side effects to expect, and how to report them promptly.

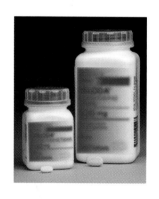

OTHER SIDE EFFECTS

Some of the less-frequent side effects of chemotherapy can include mouth sores and intestinal problems.

The mouth, stomach, and intestines are lined with cells that divide relatively rapidly. Anti-cancer drugs can affect these organs, leading to mouth sores and diarrhea.

It is a good idea to see your dentist before you begin chemotherapy to take care of any preexisting problems such as cavities or abscesses. Ask your dentist to advise you on how to brush and floss during chemotherapy.

Maintaining good mouth care and using a soft toothbrush will help minimize sores. If sores do develop, you may find that frozen juices, ice cream, and watermelon can be very soothing.

Sexual Side Effects—Physical

Chemotherapy often suppresses a woman's ovarian function, reducing the amount of estrogen in the body, and causing menopause-like symptoms such as hot flashes and vaginal dryness.

Ask your doctor or nurse to recommend a suitable non-estrogen treatment to help reduce hot flashes. Use a vaginal lubricant if necessary to manage any discomfort during intercourse. To help prevent infection, avoid oil-based lubricants such as petroleum jelly, wear cotton underwear and pantyhose with a ventilated cotton lining, and don't wear tight slacks or shorts.

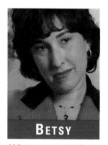

BETSY

What seems to happen a lot of times with chemo, just like with menopause, is that your vagina shrinks and shortens. And you can have problems with dryness. That's the straw that breaks the camel's back sometimes. It's too embarrassing to even think about, let alone talk to anybody.

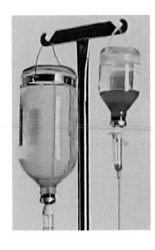

Doctors advise women of childbearing age to use birth control throughout their treatment, because anti-cancer drugs may cause birth defects. If a woman is pregnant when her cancer is discovered, it may be possible to delay chemotherapy until after the baby is born, or until after the twelfth week of pregnancy, when the fetus is beyond the stage of greatest risk.

Chemotherapy may also result in infertility. If a woman is young, and would like to have children after cancer treatment, it is now possible to harvest eggs from her ovaries, and preserve them by freezing. After treatment, the eggs can be fertilized in vitro and implanted into the woman's womb.

Egg harvesting is a difficult procedure, and may delay chemotherapy. In addition, the hormones used in harvesting and the hormonal changes due to the pregnancy may have undesirable effects on the breast cancer. Discuss these serious issues with your physician.

Sexual Side Effects—Psychological

During cancer treatment, many women find that their sexual interest declines because of the physical and emotional stresses. Don't be shy about discussing sexual issues with your nurse or doctor. They can offer a wealth of advice on how to handle any difficulties you may be facing, and help improve your quality of life.

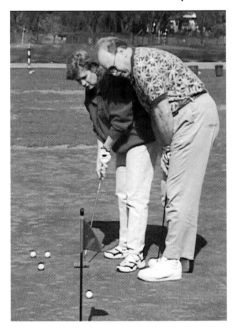

If you and your partner find it difficult to talk to each other about sex, or cancer, or both, you may want to seek out a counselor who can help you communicate more openly.

In Chapter 13 of this book we will discuss in greater detail how you can deal with this issue.

Oral care during cancer treatment:

If you develop sores in your mouth, be sure to contact your doctor or nurse because you may need medical treatment for the sores. If the sores are painful or keep you from eating, you also can try these ideas:

- Eat foods cold or at room temperature. Hot and warm foods can irritate a tender mouth and throat.
- Choose soft, soothing foods, such as ice cream, milkshakes, baby food, soft fruits (bananas and apple sauce), mashed potatoes, cooked cereals, soft-boiled or scrambled eggs, macaroni and cheese, custards, and puddings. You also can puree cooked foods in the blender to make them smoother and easier to eat.
- Avoid irritating, acidic foods, such as tomatoes, or citrus fruit (orange, grapefruit, and lemon); spicy or salty foods; and rough, coarse, or dry foods such as raw vegetables, granola, and toast.

If mouth dryness bothers you or makes it hard for you to eat, try these tips:

- Ask your doctor if you should use an artificial saliva product to moisten your mouth.
- Drink plenty of liquids.
- Suck on ice chips, popsicles, or sugarless hard candy. You can also chew sugarless gum.
- Moisten dry foods with butter, margarine, gravy or sauce.
- Dunk crisp, dry foods in mild liquids.
- Use lip balm if your lips become dry.

When chemotherapy affects the lining of the intestine, the result may be diarrhea. You can try to eat smaller portions more often, and avoid high fiber foods.

Do not take any over-the-counter medications unless specifically recommended by your health care provider.

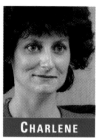

CHARLENE

I did have some trouble with mouth sores that usually set in about a week after my chemotherapy started. I got a lot of benefit from some oral swabs and a soft toothbrush.

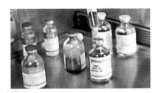

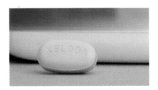

COMMON CHEMOTHERAPY DRUGS

There are dozens of drugs currently used for breast cancer treatment. Most are used in combinations of two, three, or more. Don't be confused because your doctor, nurse and pharmacist may refer to the drugs by different names. Generic name is the chemical name of the drug. Brand name is the name each manufacturer gives to their specific form of the same chemical. For example, the chemical compound called fluorouracil (its generic name) is marketed as 5-FU by one company, and as Adrucil by another. In pill form, it is known as Xeloda.

In the space below, you may want to write in specific details about the drugs that you will be taking.

CHAPTER 8

Hormone Therapy

Chemotherapy uses cytotoxic drugs to kill cancer cells. By contrast, hormone therapy uses medications that prevent cancer cells from growing by changing normal body processes.

Hormones are natural chemicals produced by the body to regulate various processes such as blood sugar metabolism, bone growth, or milk production in the breasts. Hormones include such substances as adrenaline, insulin, and estrogen.

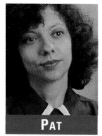

PAT

A low point was when I first started taking the hormonal therapy, because I wasn't sure how my body would react to it, but I've had no side effects, so it's gone well.

Certain types of breast cancers need the female hormones estrogen and progesterone to grow. By using chemicals that block the action of these hormones, it is possible to slow down, or even stop, the growth of cancer cells.

How exactly is this done? Some cancers are made of cells equipped with hormone receptor sites scattered over their surface. Hormone molecules fit into these sites like keys into locks, and stimulate the cells to divide. This makes the tumor grow faster. These types of cancers are called estrogen or progesterone receptor positive.

Hormone therapies work by one of three ways.

Some hormone therapies, such as the drug tamoxifen, attempt to block the effects of the hormones that the body produces. Individual molecules

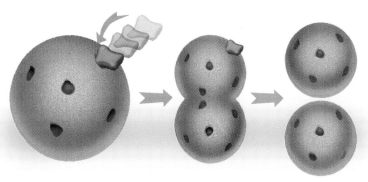

Estrogen fits into receptor sites and stimulates cell division

91

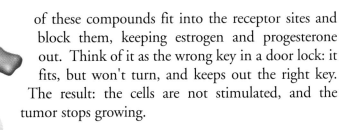

Hormonal agents block estrogen binding sites

of these compounds fit into the receptor sites and block them, keeping estrogen and progesterone out. Think of it as the wrong key in a door lock: it fits, but won't turn, and keeps out the right key. The result: the cells are not stimulated, and the tumor stops growing.

Others, such as drugs called aromatase inhibitors, keep the body from producing the hormones in the first place. Aromatase is a natural enzyme that helps produce estrogen in the woman's body. Inhibiting this enzyme can be a very effective way of reducing estrogen. Femara, Arimidex, and Aromasin are some of the aromatase inhibitors currently approved by the FDA. Estrogen and progesterone production can also be inhibited by surgically removing the ovaries.

Yet other, newer, compounds (for example, Faslodex) work by eliminating the hormone receptors on the surface of the cells, making the cells insensitive to the growth-enhancing effect of hormones.

Do not confuse hormone therapy for treatment of breast cancer, with hormone replacement therapy, or HRT, for management of hot flashes and other symptoms during menopause. Different drugs, different goals.

HOW HORMONE THERAPY IS GIVEN

As with chemotherapy, your hormone therapy should be supervised by a medical oncologist—a board-certified specialist, trained in treating cancer with drugs.

Hormone therapy is generally given in the form of a pill, although some, such as Faslodex are given as an intramuscular injection.

Who Should be Treated?

Cancer that is confined to the breast area can be treated effectively with surgery and radiation therapy. Cancer that has spread to areas beyond the breast is much more difficult to treat. Unfortunately, it is not always possible to determine with certainty at the time of diagnosis whether the cancer has spread or not.

Because of this, many clinicians recommend treatment with adjuvant, or additional therapy such as chemotherapy or hormonal therapy, or both, whenever there is a reasonable chance that cancer cells have metastasized to other parts of the body. The reasoning is that while hormone therapy and chemotherapy may be unpleasant, cancer recurrences can be life-threatening. Therefore the benefits outweigh the side effects.

Not all types of breast cancer can be treated with hormone therapy. To determine if hormone therapy is right for you, a sample of your tumor will be sent to a special lab, where it will be tested for estrogen receptors and progesterone receptors. If the tests show that your tumor is estrogen receptor positive (ER+) or progesterone receptor positive (PR+), it means that the tumor can be stimulated by these hormones. In this case, your medical oncologist may recommend hormone therapy. If the tests are negative, hormone therapy will have no effect on the growth of your cancer, regardless of your age.

SIDE EFFECTS OF HORMONE THERAPY

The side effects of hormone therapy vary with the type of therapy used. In general, hormone therapy has far fewer, and less severe, side effects than chemotherapy.

Because hormone therapy blocks estrogen, it may cause the same symptoms as going through menopause, including hot flashes, changes in menstrual periods and vaginal dryness.

Hormone therapy may affect the rate of loss of calcium from bones, which may lead to osteoporosis. Ask your physician if you need to have a simple test called bone densitometry to determine whether your bones are in danger of becoming too brittle.

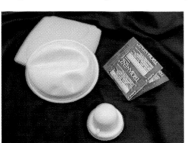
Barrier contraceptives

While you are on hormone therapy, you may still get pregnant, even if your periods have stopped as a result of the treatment. Since hormone therapy may be harmful to the fetus, it's important to use birth con-

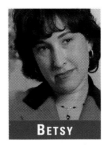
BETSY

In my case, my doctors did not recommend tamoxifen because my hormone receptors were negative. It's actually the one test that's good to hear is positive.

QUESTIONS TO ASK YOUR DOCTOR:

☐ **What side effects should I expect?**

☐ **Can I get pregnant while taking tamoxifen?**

☐ **What birth control method would be most suitable to my lifestyle?**

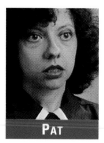

PAT

I would like to have children. Two doctors have said "No," and one has said it's OK. So, we're in limbo right now. If the hormone receptors were negative, there would be no problem with getting pregnant.

trol if you are sexually active. Do not use an oral contraceptive, or an injection or implant that contains hormones, since they may interfere with your hormone therapy. Instead, use a barrier method, such as a condom or a diaphragm.

Feel free to discuss with your doctor or nurse any sexual difficulties that you may be experiencing due to hormone therapy. Remember, there are many ways of helping you maintain your sexual activity even while you are being treated. In Chapter 13 we will review the sexual side effects of cancer therapy in greater detail.

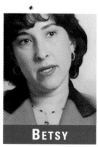

BETSY

The hardest part was thinking that I was going to lose not just my breast, but my sexuality too. Hot flashes, vaginal driness. Yuk. But once the treatment got started, I figured out how to deal with that. It was small price to pay for my life.

CHAPTER 9

Immunotherapy

Chemotherapy drugs work by attacking all fast-growing cells in the body. This approach is effective against cancer cells, but unfortunately it also damages some of the rapidly multiplying normal cells. By contrast, immunotherapy (also called biological response modifier therapy, or biotherapy) is a relatively new approach to cancer treatment that targets cancer cells specifically.

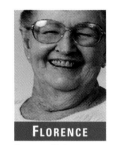

FLORENCE

I was a little concerned about this new form of therapy, but once I learned more about it, I was happy to take advantage of it.

The action of immunotherapy centers around the body's own built-in defense system—the immune system. This system includes various white blood cells (B cells, T cells, Natural Killer cells and monocytes), that circulate through the blood, each with its own specific way of attacking foreign particles, defective cells, and cancer cells. Think of the immune system as an army that relies on tanks, planes and foot soldiers, each group with its own responsibilities.

Immunotherapy works in a variety of ways:

- It can boost the immune system's natural cancer-fighting ability.

- It can coat the surface of cancer cells, cutting off the oxygen and nutrients they need to grow.

- It can make cancer cells more recognizable, and therefore more susceptible to destruction.

- It can boost the killing power of your immune system cells, such as T cells, NK cells, and macrophages.

How Herceptin works

About 25% to 30% of breast cancer patients have cells that suffer from an excess of a protein called HER-2/neu. This causes the cells to grow faster, and make tumors that are more aggressive. Herceptin finds and attaches itself to the HER-2/neu protein on the surface of these cells, slowing their growth. There is little if any effect on normal cells, which do not have an excess of HER-2/neu. Herceptin also works by attracting the body's own immune cells to help them find and destroy the cancer cells.

HERCEPTIN

For a long time, scientists have been looking for new drugs that could tell the difference between normal and cancerous cells. The search is beginning to bear results.

The first immunotherapy compound to gain acceptance in breast cancer treatment is called Herceptin. Herceptin is a monoclonal antibody. An antibody is a protein naturally produced by the body to fight off all foreign particles. A monoclonal antibody is a protein bioengineered in a laboratory and designed to target certain cancer cells.

Who can benefit from Herceptin treatment?

After the biopsy, your tumor will be tested for a variety of items, including the protein HER-2/neu. The tumor can be tested at a later date, if the biopsy sample was saved by the hospital. If the cells show an excess of HER-2/neu, chances are you will benefit from treatment with Herceptin. A new test, using serum rather than tissue, can monitor the patient's response to treatment, in real time.

Currently Herceptin is FDA-approved for use in select women whose advanced breast cancer has spread to other parts of the body, but scientists are investigating its effectiveness in early breast cancer also.

SIDE EFFECTS OF IMMUNOTHERAPY

Even though immunotherapy is more focused on abnormal cells than either chemotherapy or hormone therapy, it still causes some unwanted side effects. One example is flu-like symptoms after the first injections. In addition, Herceptin may interfere with the effective pumping of the heart, so the oncologist may order periodic MUGA scans of the heart to assess its function.

Even so, the side effects of immunotherapy are far less severe than the ones caused by chemotherapy.

FUTURE THERAPIES

Many experts believe that Herceptin represents the future direction of breast cancer drugs, because it targets a particular protein on the cancer cell, rather than attacking all cells at random. As research progresses, scientists hope to make all anti-cancer drugs as specific as possible.

QUESTIONS TO ASK YOUR DOCTOR:

☐ Is immunotherapy right for me?

☐ Would I benefit more from chemotherapy or hormonal therapy?

CHAPTER 10

Complementary and Alternative Therapies

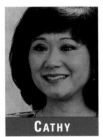

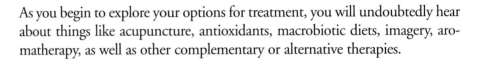

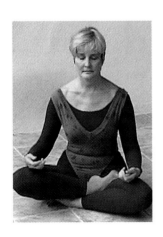

CATHY

Remember spiritually, psychologically, emotionally, that fighting this disease is multi-faceted and treat this disease within you that way. Treat every aspect of it with everything that you've got.

As you begin to explore your options for treatment, you will undoubtedly hear about things like acupuncture, antioxidants, macrobiotic diets, imagery, aromatherapy, as well as other complementary or alternative therapies.

It's extremely important that you understand the difference between so-called conventional or traditional medicine, and complementary or alternative therapies.

Conventional treatment is what is currently accepted by reputable healthcare providers. It is based on decades of sound medical research, and represents the best that Western medicine has to offer today.

Complementary treatments may or may not have been rigorously evaluated. They are widely and successfully used to relieve side effects of cancer treatment, and to enhance the quality of life.

Alternative therapies, by contrast, have no medically sound foundation, and represent a dangerous temptation for those who may be skeptical about traditional medical treatment.

Consult your healthcare team before trying any type of complementary therapy to make sure it won't interfere with your treatment. And certainly have an informed discussion with them if you are contemplating embarking on an alternative course of treatment.

COMPLEMENTARY THERAPIES

Practitioners refer to these therapies as complementary, rather than alternative, because they are to be used only in conjunction with—not instead of—

the treatment recommended by your doctors. You still need surgery, or chemotherapy or whatever other conventional treatment is right for you.

There is a wide variety of complementary techniques, some based on principles adopted from other specialties (for example, relaxation), from Oriental medicine (acupuncture) from Indian medicine (yoga), or even from ancient Egyptian culture (aromatherapy.)

Mind/Body Connection

Many complementary therapies are based on the principle of mind/body connection. For centuries, people have believed that there is a connection between the state of the mind and the health of the body. How this connection worked, however, was never quite clear.

Recently, scientists have identified chemicals, called neurotransmitters, by which nerve cells communicate with one another. Neurotransmitters are also involved in the control of emotions. For example, antidepressant medications increase the amount of norepinephrine and serotonin in the spaces between nerve cells. These same neurotransmitters have effects elsewhere in the body, affecting heart rate and blood pressure, and may even influence the activity of cells in the immune system.

Changes in the state of the nervous system which can occur because of stress or lack of social support, can influence many organ systems. For example, it has been found that people under stress are more likely to develop colds.

Anxiety, grief, stress, and fear of the unknown all seem to have an impact on the body. Learning to cope with these emotions, using a wide variety of approaches—such as meditation and visualization, spiritual support, and participation in support groups—may help speed your recovery, and benefit your health.

Meditation and Visualization

Meditation has been shown to produce physiological responses such as a decrease in blood pressure, respiration rate, and overall metabolism—all of which contribute to reducing stress on our minds and bodies. Guided imagery or visualization (for example, visualizing natural killer cells gobbling up cancers cells like in the game Pac-Man) can also be used with meditation.

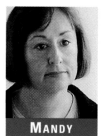

MANDY

I listened to tapes by Bernie Siegel, read motivational literature and practical self-hypnosis books. I took vitamins, especially C, E, and beta carotene. I rode my exercise bike almost daily. When I felt weak , I napped and tried not to feel guilty about sleeping during the day. I believe all these therapies were an important part of my recovery.

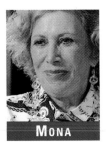

MONA

*I immediately started medi-
tation and guided imagery.
I went to see a woman, a
psychiatrist, who had had a
double mastectomy and was
very understanding of the
problems that I was going
through. I felt that I needed
to let out a lot of rage and
hostility in a controlled
environment.*

There is no claim that meditation and visualization cure cancer, but studies have proven that a combination of these techniques can reduce pain and other uncomfortable side effects of cancer treatment.

To demystify the terms "meditation" and "visualization", many physicians simply refer to these techniques as "stress reduction," or "relaxation."

Spiritual Support

Since prehistoric times, prayer has been one of the most common ways of dealing with pain and illness in all civilizations. Today many accept that some form of spiritual support is a basic human need. Prayer, laying on of hands, and many forms of spiritual imagery or inner dialogue have helped patients find the higher strength within themselves to cope with breast cancer and other illness.

Many cancer patients rely on their spiritual experiences and established religious traditions to regain control and gather additional strength to battle cancer. Even those who have little or no connection with religion often find themselves moved by the "spiritual emergency" of cancer.

Humor / Laughter

Laughter can stimulate endorphins—chemicals that act like opiates in the brain. You might find humor and laughter emotionally healing. In addition, giving yourself time not to think about your cancer can have a wonderfully invigorating effect.

While some enjoy standup comedians, others may prefer Marx Brothers movies or sitcom reruns, such as "I Love Lucy." While undergoing cancer treatment, writer Norman Cousins discovered that ten minutes of genuine belly laughter had an anesthetic effect that would give him at least two hours of pain-free sleep.

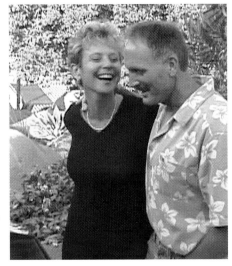

Diet

There's still a great deal of controversy on the subject of nutrition and its effect on breast cancer. So far, there's no scientific data to prove one diet better than another for breast cancer treatment, although there is some evidence that a low fat diet may decrease the incidence of recurrence of breast cancer in post-menopausal women.

Most physicians recommend that patients simply follow good nutrition, with particular emphasis on protein and vitamins during chemotherapy treatment. A consultation with a nutritionist will help you learn more about your particular needs.

Macrobiotic diets emphasize whole grains, miso soup, fresh vegetables and beans, with little fruit and no sugar. Special diets such as these may someday prove to be effective for patients with certain types of cancer, but more scientific research is needed in this area.

Herbal Therapy

The majority of herbal therapies are based on the belief that they improve organ function. There is increasing evidence from Asian and European countries that some herbs can be effective in fighting cancer. Common herbs and medicinal plants used for breast cancer include Astragalus root, burdock root, garlic, green tea, licorice root and a variety of others.

Some herbal preparations are extremely potent and may be harmful. Practitioners should dispense herbs on an individualized basis in accordance with each patient's needs. You should always consult your healthcare professional before beginning herbal therapy, since some preparations may interfere with your treatment.

Vitamins

Many biological processes in the body lead to the formation of toxic products such as toxic lipid peroxides, which can damage DNA in cells, leading to cancer. Vitamins C, E, and beta-carotene are "anti-oxidant" vitamins commonly used to neutralize these potentially toxic products. In addition, elements such as selenium and copper may be useful, in trace amounts only, to facilitate the defense against toxic peroxides.

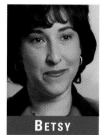

BETSY

I got back into meditation, into bio-feedback, into guided imagery. I cleaned up my diet, took the vitamins that I needed to take, and the herbs, and looked into acupuncture and some other modalities. And I think it really enhanced the way I dealt with chemo. I never threw up. I never lost all of my hair, though I was told that I would.

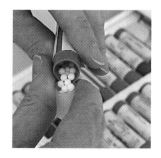

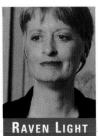

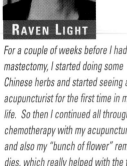

For a couple of weeks before I had my mastectomy, I started doing some Chinese herbs and started seeing an acupuncturist for the first time in my life. So then I continued all through my chemotherapy with my acupuncture and also my "bunch of flower" remedies, which really helped with the terror of going for chemotherapy.

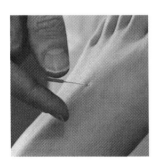

It is generally thought by radiation oncologists that antioxidants may interfere with the beneficial effects of radiation, and should be used only with the approval of your radiation oncologist.

Talk with your physician or nutritionist, or contact the National Cancer Institure or the American Cancer Society to find out about the latest recommendations on the topic of antioxidants and vitamins.

OTHER COMPLEMENTARY THERAPIES

Acupuncture and homeopathy are based on the concept that there is a life force within our body organs. This life force—an animating factor—maintains the body in a state of health, and predisposes us to disease when it is unbalanced.

Acupuncture

Acupuncture is a technique, first developed in ancient China, which involves insertion and manipulation of needles at specific points in the body to balance the life force.

The theory behind acupuncture is that there are special meridian points on the body that are connected to internal organs. Vital energy flows along the meridian lines, and diseases are caused by an imbalance of this flow. Normal flow of vital energy is restored by inserting needles at the meridian points. Current research studies suggest that acupuncture needles may work by triggering the release of natural pain inhibitors.

In China, acupuncture has long been used for pain relief, and for treatment of ailments such as arthritis, hypertension, and ulcers. It is now also used as anesthesia during childbirth and some types of surgery. Acupuncture has been used with some success by a number of Western physicians, to relieve nausea, pain or other symptoms associated with cancer.

Homeopathy

Practitioners of homeopathy believe that minute, highly diluted doses of a medicine treat the life force—not the physical force—of organs such as the liver, kidneys, or intestines. Although homeopathy is questioned by most American physicians, it is widely used in Europe and Asia.

ALTERNATIVE TREATMENTS

Reputable medical practitioners believe that before anything can be safely used as a treatment, it must undergo rigorous testing and evaluation, using large numbers of patients, and objective analysis of the results.

But from time to time, a new product suddenly appears, and is promoted as the new alternative to standard medical treatment for cancer. Most of the time, the claims are founded on a few poorly documented cases of alleged "cures," and sometimes on nothing but a promoter's greed or ignorance.

An example is laetril—a substance made from apricot pits, that was presented as a cure for cancer, based on the claim that cyanide contained in the apricot pits killed cancer cells. Scientific studies, and personal experiences of patients who tried the treatment on their own, have proven laetril to be useless or even harmful, and there have been reports of deaths from cyanide poisoning.

Tips for Evaluating False Claims

When considering use of alternative therapies, it is important to balance promotional information provided by sellers with objective, evidence-based information that you can obtain from your healthcare provider.

- The product is advertised as a quick and effective cure-all.

- The promoters use words like scientific breakthrough, miraculous cure, exclusive product, secret ingredient or ancient remedy.

- The promoter claims the government, the medical profession or research scientists have conspired to suppress the product.

- The advertisement includes undocumented amazing results.

- The product is advertised as available from only one source, and payment is required in advance.

- The promoter promises a no-risk "money-back guarantee." Many won't be around to respond to your request for a refund.

QUESTIONS TO ASK:

- [ ] **What benefits can be expected from this therapy?**

- [ ] **What are the risks associated with this therapy?**

- [ ] **Do the known benefits outweigh the risks?**

- [ ] **What side effects can be expected?**

- [ ] **Will the therapy interfere with conventional treatment?**

- [ ] **Will the therapy be covered by health insurance?**

DCIS

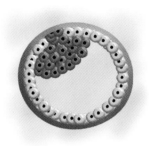

In situ cancer

This chapter deals with DCIS—*ductal carcinoma in situ*—a very early, non-invasive breast cancer classified as Stage 0. If you were diagnosed with a higher stage of cancer, you may skip this chapter.

WHAT IS DCIS?

DCIS is a ductal cancer that has not yet penetrated the lining of the duct. In other words, it is not invasive. In this *in situ* ("in place") stage, the cancer has not spread into the blood stream and beyond. If it is diagnosed and treated correctly, the risk of dying from this cancer is essentially zero.

In the past, DCIS was rare—most breast cancers were found when the tumor had grown large enough to be felt by hand. By then it had time to spread outside the breast. But with the increased use of mammography in the past 20 years, DCIS has become relatively easy to detect. It appears on mammograms as a speckling of tiny white dots—clumps of dead cancer cells that became calcified inside the ducts. Today, about 20-30% of cancers diagnosed are DCIS. Still, in comparison to invasive cancers, it has not had the time to be researched as extensively, and there is some disagreement among physicians as to how to treat it.

MASTECTOMY OR LUMPECTOMY?

Until recently, it was firmly believed that the best way to treat DCIS was to perform a simple mastectomy. The feeling was that since the cancer has not yet spread (remember, DCIS is in situ!) all one had to do was remove the breast for essentially a 100% guarantee of cure.

As lumpectomy plus radiation became an acceptable choice for invasive breast cancer, surgeons learned that if they removed a small DCIS tumor with a wide margin around it and treated the breast with radiation, they can achieve a much nicer cosmetic result. But that comes at the expense of a small chance of future local cancer recurrence. The decision is up to the patient and her healthcare provider.

RADIATION THERAPY OR NOT?

The other area where there may be a difference of opinion is radiation therapy. This is where DCIS treatment differs from treatment of early invasive breast cancer. A Stage I or II tumor treated with breast conserving surgery—lumpectomy—will always be treated with radiation too.

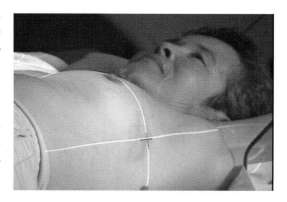

But some specialists believe that there is no need for radiating the breast if the DCIS tumor was small, and the margins were large and clear—in other words, if there is a fair degree of certainty that the tumor was indeed *in situ*.

The reason to avoid radiating a breast after a surgical excision of a DCIS tumor, is that if the cancer does recur, the patient will no longer have the option of breast conserving surgery. Since radiation therapy can be used only once on the same area of the body, the next time, treatment will require a mastectomy, rather than a lumpectomy. This is another dilemma that requires discussion with your healthcare team.

Beam alignment for radiation therapy

TREATMENT OF DCIS

To make the decisions easier, researchers devised a system for selecting the best treatment plan for each DCIS lesion. It is based on the size of the tumor, the grade of the tumor cells, and the width of the margins around the tumor.

Before surgery, an accurate mammogram is obtained, to determine exactly the size and shape of the DCIS lesion.

The surgeon removes the tumor with a large margin of normal tissue, striving for at least a half inch on all sides.

The radiologist takes an X-ray of the tissue removed and compares it with the original mammogram, to ensure that the entire tumor was removed. Immediately after the X-ray, while the patient is still in the operating room, a pathologist makes numerous slices across the tumor and examines each slice in detail. Applying black ink to the outside of the tumor makes it easier to determine if the margins are "clear."

If the tumor was small, the grade of the cells was low, and the margins were at least 10mm (less than half an inch) there is no need for removing additional tissue, or for radiation therapy.

If the tumor was larger, the cells more aggressive, or the margins too narrow, then the DCIS tumor may be treated with a simple mastectomy, or lumpectomy with radiation.

YOUR TEAM

If you were diagnosed with DCIS, you may consider investing some time into finding a medical center with an experienced team—a surgeon, a pathologist and a mammographer who work well together in assessing in situ tumors. In this way you will be assured of the best chances for a successful treatment, with the least loss of breast tissue.

CHAPTER 12

Clinical Trials

WHAT ARE TRIALS?

Scientists are constantly searching for better ways of dealing with breast cancer. Many women diagnosed with breast cancer may benefit from this research by participating in clinical trials.

A clinical trial is an evaluation of a new way of managing cancer. Some trials are designed to see if a new drug or a new procedure will be effective in treating or preventing cancer. Other trials evaluate new ways to diagnose the disease. Still others concentrate on finding a new way to eliminate unwanted side effects.

Clinical trials help improve the quality of care, now and in the future. One such trial, conducted many years ago, showed that lumpectomy with radiation treatment was as effective as removal of the entire breast, which was the standard practice back then. As a result of this trial, many women today can enjoy the benefits of breast-conserving surgery.

Clinical trials are not random attempts to discover something new. Trials are conducted according to very specific guidelines that are recognized by the medical community worldwide. By ensuring uniformity, it is possible to be confident that results obtained in one location, will be readily comparable to results from another location, even in another country.

New treatments are first tested in laboratories, using animals. Animal research offers scientists the only way to make the transition from something that works in a test tube to something that will work in people, without risking human lives unnecessarily in the process.

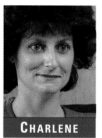

CHARLENE

When the word "research" was first presented to me, I felt very fearful: Is this something that's only been tried on me? Am I the research rat? But when I learned more, I realized that it wasn't like that. I felt very fortunate knowing that I was getting aggressive therapy and that I would only benefit from it.

If there is initial evidence that the treatment may be effective, it is then evaluated further with actual patients, usually with advanced stages of the disease.

To reach the next trial stage, where large numbers of patients are used, the treatment method or drug must have demonstrated that it offers potential benefit, without unacceptable risk.

If the clinical trial confirms the benefits, the drug or treatment will be made available to all patients.

HOW ARE TRIALS CONDUCTED?

Every trial is conducted according to a protocol—a set of guidelines that spells out exactly what will be done and when. Large numbers of patients are selected according to very specific criteria—age, stage of cancer, previous treatment, and so forth.

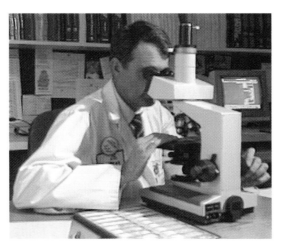

The patients who meet these criteria are enrolled into the study, and divided into groups. Most trials consist of a control group (patients who are receiving standard therapy) and a treatment group (those who receive the new therapy that is being evaluated.) The treatment group always receives treatment that is considered to be at least as good, and possibly better, than the standard treatment. Sometimes the control group receives a placebo—an injection or a pill that looks like the drug being evaluated, but has no medicinal value; for example, a sugar pill instead of a drug.

Patients are assigned to one of the two groups by a random, computerized system, where neither the patient nor the physician has control over the selection. In addition, neither the patient nor the investigator knows which group the patient was placed in, until the end of the trial. This process is called double-blind randomization. The purpose is to avoid bias on the part of the patient or the treating physician. In other words, random assignment keeps the researcher from favoring one or the other group, and skewing the results. Not knowing whether the actual drug or a placebo is being administered, eliminates pre-concieved notions, and keeps the patient from reporting improvement or side effects that may be imaginary.

A central agency keeps all the records of the selection, and can reveal them if the need arises. Sometimes, if one group is showing a significantly better response than the other, the trial is terminated, and all patients are given the better treatment.

PARTICIPATING IN A TRIAL

If your physician does not mention trials, you may want to bring up the subject on your own. There are many trials going on around the country, and you may just find one that matches your case perfectly.

Generally, you or your physician can obtain information about ongoing trials from the National Cancer Institute's hotline called PDQ, or from the local chapter of the American Cancer Society.

You and your physician will review the lists of requirements for various trials to see whether or not you might qualify for one of them. If you do, be sure to find out what is involved in terms of tests, treatments, additional time commitments, and side effects, and evaluate whether or not you can live with these terms for an extended time. Then assess the possible benefits to you, and balance them against the negatives.

If you decide to proceed, you will be asked to sign an informed consent form, to show that you understand the issues involved, the expected benefits, the possible side effects, your rights and responsibilities, and the possible outcome.

You will be asked to follow the schedule of treatments and tests as closely as possible, in order to make the information obtained scientifically sound.

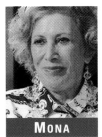

MONA

When I was asked to be on a research study, it was very carefully explained to me by my doctor and his nurse. I took a copy of the papers home, and as a matter of fact, sent one to a female physician friend of mine. We talked on the phone about it. I felt that I would be carefully watched and carefully monitored. So I had no hesitation.

IS A TRIAL RIGHT FOR ME?

Trials are what makes it possible for medicine to make progress. But you won't be participating purely for the good of others. Being part of a trial offers a definite benefit for you personally, whether you are assigned to the treatment group and receive the new drug, or you windup in the control group and receive conventional therapy.

One of the advantages of being in a clinical trial is that patients in both treatment and control groups enjoy a higher standard of care, because trial protocols usually call for more frequent tests, more frequent visits to the hospital, and more thorough examinations.

And there are few, if any, downsides. Your participation is completely optional and voluntary. You can leave the trial at any time. If you drop out, you will not be penalized in any way, and you will still be entitled to the best standard treatment available.

CHAPTER 13

Life After Cancer

You had your last dose of chemotherapy, or your last radiation treatment. The surgical scars are beginning to heal. As your energy and confidence return, you'll be able to explore the many options for moving forward from the cancer experience, to a new life.

EMOTIONAL RECOVERY

A diagnosis of cancer impacts your self-esteem, your body image, your sexuality—even your outlook on survival. You probably realize that life will never be the same after such an experience. This will leave you with a sense of loss. Take time to grieve the loss. This grieving process is an important first step toward the healing of the mind.

Reactive Depression

As you try to come to terms with your diagnosis and try to deal with the impact of your treatment, you are likely to have episodes of anxiety and depression. It is important for you to be able to distinguish depression that you can cope with on your own, from depression that requires professional help.

As is the case for most women undergoing cancer treatment, there will be times when you are sad—times when you are "feeling blue." This is called reactive depression—in other words, you are having an appropriate reaction to your situation. This level of depression is normal, and most women can cope with it, with help from family, friends, or support groups.

QUESTIONS TO ASK YOUR DOCTOR OR NURSE:

☐ What can I do if I wake up at night worrying about my cancer?

☐ Will the cancer cells that may have spread to other parts of my body start to grow when I stop taking chemotherapy?

☐ Should my sisters get genetically tested?

☐ Shouldn't we be doing more testing on me to make sure the cancer didn't come back?

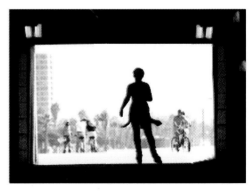

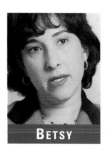

BETSY

At least while I was in chemotherapy, I was actually doing something to take charge of the cancer, to kill any cancer cells that might be running amuck in my body. When I walked out of the chemo suite for the last time, there was a feeling of, "Now what? Where do I go from here?"

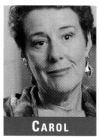

CAROL

I found it really important to learn to laugh at myself. The whole thing is a disaster, and if you can find some little bits of humor in it, you might feel better. Remember, the universe is proceeding exactly the way it's supposed to be, whatever happens to you. So you just put one foot in front of the other and do the things that need to be done.

One method that helps manage anxiety and depression is planning pleasant activities such as going out with friends or seeing a movie around the times when you normally feel depressed.

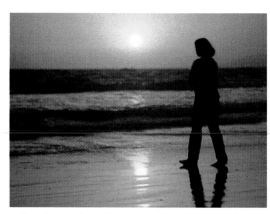

Another approach is exercise and sports. Physical activity stimulates the body to produce certain chemicals called endorphins that help restore a sense of well being. Try to get out of your mind and into your body, so to speak.

Other effective techniques include relaxation and visualization, described in the chapter on Complementary Therapies.

If you haven't already, consider joining a support group. You should have no trouble finding one that matches your lifestyle and your particular needs. You will find a list of resources for referral to support groups at the end of the book.

There are specific times during the course of treatment and recovery when bouts of anxiety and depression are more likely to occur.

Most women experience their highest level of anxiety when they come home from the hospital after surgery, because coming home means leaving most of the medical team behind and resuming normal activities.

Another time women may feel anxious or depressed is when their chemotherapy or radiation treatments end. There may be a feeling of panic at the thought that you are not being treated any more. This post-treatment anxiety is quite natural, and will gradually diminish as you regain confidence.

Some women notice that they are particularly anxious on the anniversary dates of their diagnosis or surgery. These are the so-called anniversary reactions. In addition, many women also may have "check up anxiety" just before their scheduled follow-up visit to the physician.

Clinical Depression

There is a form of depression that is unlikely to improve on its own. Usually it includes continuous feelings of sadness, feelings of worthlessness or guilt, excessive fear of the future, and lack of interest in intimacy or sex. This is called clinical depression and requires intervention by a trained professional.

Clinical depression can be treated. It may involve counseling, medications, and perhaps physical exercise and stress reduction techniques. Your physician will be able to refer you to the appropriate specialist.

And remember, you should never feel embarrassed to seek professional help. It is not a sign of weakness—no more so than going to a surgeon for a lumpectomy. Most cases of depression are short, and usually respond to counseling, with or without the use of some of the very effective medications available today.

You may have a clinical depression if you:

- Are continuously sad for weeks
- Withdraw from friends and relatives
- Feel worthless
- Fear the future excessively
- Speak or move slowly
- Feel tired all the time
- Can't make decisions
- Are angry all the time
- Lost interest in intimacy and sex

If you experience several of these symptoms, you should discuss your situation with your physician. If you have thoughts about suicide, call your physician or nurse immediately.

PHYSICAL RECOVERY

Regular Follow-Up

Even after the most complete treatment, there's always a chance that cancer will recur. Most recurrences happen two or three years after surgery. The longer you go without a recurrence, the greater are your chances of remain-

QUESTIONS TO ASK YOUR DOCTOR OR NURSE:

☐ What can I do about feeling excessively tired?

☐ Why have I lost interest in intimate relations with my partner?

☐ Why can't I sleep or relax or feel interested in anything?

☐ Why can't I stop feeling that I am going to die because of the cancer?

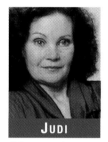

JUDI

A few months ago, my son and I went for a trip to the Grand Canyon, and that's something I've always wanted to do. Just getting out and taking photographs, seeing new and different parts of the country, I felt much, much better than if I had just stayed at home feeling sorry for myself. And I find that if my attitude is positive I do feel much better than if I allow myself to become depressed.

ing free of disease. But you can never say that the cancer has been completely cured.

Because of this possibility, you need regular follow-up visits with a healthcare professional. It could be your family physician, your oncologist, or your

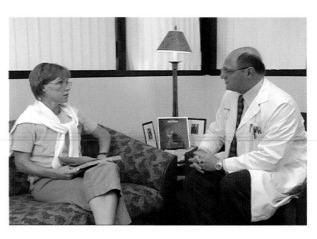

breast surgeon. What's important is to have a single person in charge of the follow-up care. Usually you'll be seen as often as every few weeks immediately after treatment, and perhaps only every six months later on. There is no "right" schedule. Eventually, you will probably be down to a single annual visit.

What does follow-up involve? Most physicians suggest a physical examination to look for signs of local recurrence—new lumps within the breast after lumpectomy, or tiny hard nodules in the surgical scar after mastectomy.

In addition, mammography will be scheduled on a regular basis, and you may have a number of blood tests that will assess the function of your liver, bone marrow, and other organs, and a chest X-ray. Other tests such as CEA (a protein found in the blood of patients with cancer) and bone scans are not used routinely.

Currently, many experts feel that there is little to be gained by performing multiple tests on patients that are asymptomatic—that is patients who have no symptoms. Such tests may detect a recurrence a few months earlier, but earlier diagnosis will not change the outcome of whatever treatment you might need.

Breast Self Examination (BSE)

One of the key components of follow-up is your monthly breast self-examination, or BSE.

Recently you might have read that BSE is not effective in saving lives. But many leading experts and patient advocacy groups remain convinced that women who are well trained in BSE should continue to examine their own breasts. BSE is particularly important for women at higher risk of breast cancer—and that includes you and your first degree relatives.

BSE is not a skill that you can learn from a brochure or a shower card. The best way to learn it is from your healthcare provider, or from a good breast self exam video. Check the Library section at the end of the book to find out how you can get the most up-to-date instructional videos on BSE.

A thorough BSE should include:

Looking: Using a mirror, check the shape and size of your breasts, and the color and texture of your skin, first with your arms down, then with your arms in the air. Try to learn what's normal for you, so that you can spot any changes immediately.

Check your breasts in two other positions—pushing down on the hips, to tighten your chest muscles, and bending forward at the waist, with your arms relaxed. This will help you spot dimpling—the tugging on the skin or nipple often caused by a growing tumor.

Next, lie down with a folded towel under your shoulder. Extend the arm out at an angle to spread the breast tissue more evenly. You will need to examine the breast as well as the area where breast tissue may be found—from the armpit, to the breast bone, and from the collar bone to the bra line.

Use three middle fingers to examine the breast. Use the pads because they're more sensitive than the tips. Keeping the fingers straight with the pads flat against the breast, make three dime-sized circles. One just lightly, one deeper, one deeper still. This will enable you to check the full thickness of your breast.

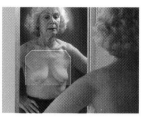

Check your breasts in the mirror

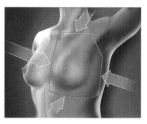

Examine the entire breast area

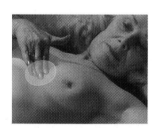

Make three little circles with your fingertips

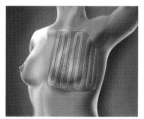

Move your fingers in vertical strips

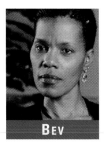

BEV

I never really understood it, but I've had so many... you know, offers... after my mastectomy, I almost think I should have had this a long time ago. It could be men are attracted to my drive to live, because I was faced with an illness that could have caused my death.

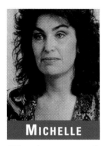

MICHELLE

It has been approximately two years since my reconstruction. I feel very much like a woman. And I don't just feel normal, I feel very attractive. I feel like I have my sexuality back and I feel that I would be attractive to any man.

When you move your hand, don't lift the fingers away from the skin, to avoid missing a spot. Cover the entire area, spot by spot, going up and down in strips about as wide as your three fingers.

When you've finished, lower your arm and examine your armpit for possible lymph node enlargement. Then check the other breast the same way.

If you had a mastectomy you are not likely to find a lump within the flap tissue used for reconstruction. Local recurrences are more likely to appear as tiny firm beads along the incision line.

If you had a lumpectomy, you will probably feel irregular lumpiness at the surgical sight shortly after the lumpectomy heals. You need to become familiar with the new look and feel of your breasts, so that you can report any changes promptly.

Clinical Breast Examination

CBE will be part of your regular check ups. The physician will probably spend additional time examining the scar and areas where enlarged lymph nodes may be found—under the arms, and around the collar bones.

Mammography

Every woman who has had breast cancer should have a mammogram once a year, regardless of age.

If you had a lumpectomy, the films may be more difficult to interpret, so make sure that previous mammograms are available for comparison.

If you had a mastectomy, you should have mammograms of the other breast. If you are sensitive near the post-surgical scar, ask the technologist for a Mammopad—a soft sheet of special padding that fits on the mammography device.

MRI

For women with especially dense breasts, or women who present unusual diagnostic challenges, MRI is often an effective although expensive option.

Care of the Surgical Arm

After a mastectomy and particularly if you also had a lymph node dissection, your arm may feel numb and tingly due to nerve damage during surgery. Later, you may feel shooting pains due to nerve re-growth. You may also have decreased range of motion or weakness in the shoulder as a result of nerve damage or as a result of prolonged disuse.

There is not much that you can do to reverse numbness due to nerve damage. Some of it may improve as the nerves heal over the years.

Your healthcare professional will tell you which exercises are appropriate to help your arm regain its mobility and strength. It is very important to follow the exercise schedule faithfully so you can recover your full range of motion. You will find a description of some of the exercises in the mastectomy section of the Surgery Chapter. Once you regain your full range of motion, you will not need to continue these exercises.

As you have read in Chapter 4, lymphedema is swelling of the arm due to scarring of the lymph ducts after surgery or radiation. This condition occurs in approximately ten to twenty women out of a hundred, sometimes months or years after surgery.

It is important that you always follow your medical team's recommendations about how to avoid injury to the arm to reduce the chances of developing lymphedema.

INTIMACY AND SEXUALITY

Your Self Image

We live in a society that considers breasts to be an important aspect of a woman's attractiveness. The loss of a breast after a mastectomy, or even a slight change in shape after a lumpectomy may have a serious impact on a woman's confidence. "Will I still be loved?" "Will I be attractive?" are valid questions that need to be answered in a woman's mind.

Doubts about your appearance and attractiveness are normal, but you should not let them affect your self-image. Remember, there is much more

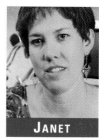

JANET

It didn't affect my sexual relationship at all. Maybe it enlightened it because I think that our love grew from the experience. It definitely didn't get worse.

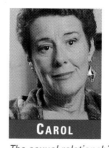

CAROL

The sexual relationships that I was in after the mastectomy required communication that hadn't been there before. I had to be able to tell people what would feel good.

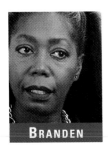

BRANDEN

I started a journal before the mastectomy, when I was first diagnosed with breast cancer. Later, I got a grant from the National Endowment for the Arts, took the journal, turned it into a play, and premiered it at the Los Angeles Theater Center.

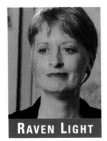

RAVEN LIGHT

I'm a highly sexual woman and so is my lover. I was scared that I would not be able to satisfy her. But my nurse helped us talk the issues out and relearn how to enjoy intimacy.

to sexuality and pleasure—and to you as a person—than the shape or presence of a breast.

The critical issue is not the loss of the breast itself, but the way you and your partner treat the loss. Open communication is very important. Many couples find to their surprise that the patient is more concerned about the loss of her breast than her partner is.

SIDE EFFECTS OF TREATMENT

The side effects of treatment will vary with the treatment choice, and with your own response.

Many of the side effects are easy to anticipate. Surgery could decrease or eliminate entirely nipple sensation—which may affect sexual arousal. Radiation therapy may render breast skin more irritable during treatment, and perhaps less sensitive years later. Overall, the emotional and physical demands of treatment take their toll, leading to fatigue. Most of these side effects are relatively short lived, or tolerable.

Other consequences of treatment may have a greater impact. For example, if you did not yet go through menopause, chemotherapy or hormonal therapy is almost certain to stop your periods—temporarily or permanently. If you are young, your periods are more likely to return than if you are approaching menopause.

Menopause caused by chemotherapy is much more sudden, and for many, more difficult than natural menopause. You may go find that you are having mood swings that are out of character for you, and blame them on your inability to deal with cancer, whereas in reality you may be the victim of severe hormonal imbalance induced by the chemotherapy or hormone therapy. Discuss your problems with your physician. Drugs like Celexa, Paxil, Prozac and others have proven very useful in dealing with menopausal symptoms.

A less recognized side effect is that chemotherapy reduces the amounts of testosterone in the body. Testosterone is generally known only as a male hormone, but it is present in small quantities in women, and is responsible for the woman's sex drive. With loss of testosterone, there is loss of libido—a side effect that often goes unnoticed, unreported, misdiagnosed, or untreated. If loss of libido becomes a problem for you and your partner, you may want to find a healthcare provider who is well versed in the management of such problems.

FERTILITY

Even in couples who have not yet had children, the urgency of dealing with breast cancer often takes precedence over plans to build a family. Sometimes rash treatment decisions are made that cannot later be reversed. For example, embarking on a course of hormone therapy or chemotherapy may lead to infertility that is not reversible. For younger couples, future fertility is one area that merits as much research as any other aspect of breast cancer treatment.

Breast cancer in itself does not rule out the possibility of having children. Many women go on to have successful pregnancies, with no adverse effect on their health or future outcome. If you're in your child-bearing years and would like to have a baby, it is very important to discuss this issue with all the physicians on your team, including your oncologist, radiation therapist, pathologist, and surgeon. Ask them to review all the details of your case—such as cancer type, degree of spread, amount of radiation you received, and so on—before advising you on whether it is safe for you to get pregnant.

Recent advances in fertility offer new options for women who must undergo treatment that is likely to render destroy the eggs in their ovaries and render them sterile.

One option is embryo freezing. For this procedure a few of the woman's eggs are surgically removed, artificially fertilized in vitro then frozen and stored for future re-implantation in the woman's uterus. This procedure has a 10-25% success rate.

Another option is removal and storage of unfertilized eggs—a good option if the woman is not in a relationship. This procedure has a lower (3%) success rate. Make sure you review all your options with a fertility expert.

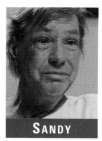

SANDY

You know, when something like this happens, then you realize what you've been missing. It's a great feeling, to walk out in the morning and smell the clean air. I never did that before.

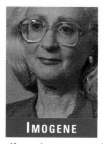

IMOGENE

If you have some talent, use it. And do something with it. Get your rage out. I think that's the most important thing for survival, and for a fuller, richer life.

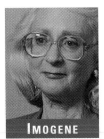

IMOGENE

Your personality isn't changed when you have breast cancer. You're the same person that you always were. If you attracted men before your breast cancer, you will attract them after your breast cancer. It'll be different, but it will be just as good.

RESUMING SEXUAL ACTIVITY

Some women and many of their partners worry about when and how it is acceptable to resume sexual activity after breast surgery. Sometimes the partner may avoid physical contact simply out of fear of causing discomfort to the woman.

There is nothing about breast surgery itself that would require a delay. Even if you still have a dressing, or drains and stitches, there is no reason not to engage in intimate contact. The decision is based more on your emotional state than on your physical readiness.

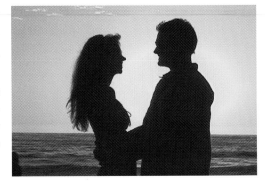

Often you will have to be one who opens the conversation about your fears or needs, because your partner may feel that these issues are too personal. Bring the subject up as early as possible. The more time passes without open discussion, the harder it becomes to deal with the issue.

If you're not ready, make it clear to your partner that not wanting to make love is not an act of rejection, and that you may welcome other forms of physical intimacy.

Some women who have had a mastectomy purchase sexy lingerie, or have intimacy in subdued lighting to help take the edge off the presence of a surgical scar, without reducing the feeling of closeness and excitement.

If you have loss of sensation in the breast or nipple area, you may need to gently guide your partner, indicating what is now pleasurable to you.

Hugging, touching, holding, and cuddling may become more important, while sexual intercourse may become less important. Remember that what was true before your cancer remains true now: There is no one "right" way to express your sexuality. It's up to you and your partner to determine together what is now pleasurable and satisfying to both of you.

SINGLE AFTER BREAST CANCER

Being single and trying to start a new relationship, while simultaneously dealing with breast cancer, can add a lot of stress to your life.

One of the challenges is deciding how and when to tell a new acquaintance, who may or may not become a love interest, that you had breast cancer.

The main obstacle is that many women who had a diagnosis of breast cancer feel that they are in some way incomplete or unworthy. "Damaged goods."

I cannot tell you how to begin a successful relationship. But I can suggest the mind-set that will guide you at least through the breast cancer issue.

The key is to realize that you are not your cancer. You are not a victim. You are not less complete, or less worthy than before your diagnosis. You are who you were. And in addition, as a result of your experience, you are now an even stronger, more interesting, and more understanding person than before. On top of that, the concept that there is something shameful about breast cancer is a thing of the past. It has been "out of the closet" for years! Just check prime time TV programming. Breast cancer is there along with other everyday issues of everyday life.

If you were diagnosed only recently, and the shock is still fresh in your mind, it is difficult if not impossible to be so confident. But have faith—soon your brain will adjust, and you will be able to put your cancer experience in perspective, and realize that it has contributed something positive to you.

How and When do I Tell Him About my Cancer?

In Chapter 1 I made a few suggestions on how to discuss your diagnosis with your life partner. But if you are starting a brand new relationship, the question is more complicated. Exactly how and when do you bring up the topic? You are not alone if the thought of informing your date that you are missing a breast makes your palms sweat.

First, how do you say it? If you are uncomfortable articulating the words, there are some tricks that may help you. You've probably heard that some

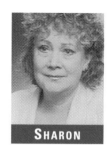

SHARON

I think one should keep up one's social interests. It's one way to fight depression. So it's important for you go out, do interesting things, maybe even things you've never done before. Push yourself a little.

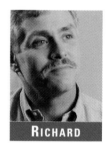

RICHARD

She had a glow about her that I found completely irresistible. Soon I found out that it was the glow of chemo, but by then I was in love…

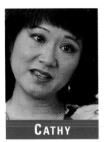

CATHY

I found it really important to learn to laugh at myself. The whole thing is a disaster, and if you can find some little bits of humor in it, you might feel better. Remember, the universe is proceeding exactly the way it's supposed to be, whatever happens to you. So you just put one foot in front of the other and do the things that need to be done.

experts recommend that if you are afraid of public speaking, just imagine that the audience is naked. So if you are afraid to say, "I had a mastectomy last year," imagine that your date is jobless, or a diabetic, or Viagra-dependent. Now who's got the sweaty palms?

Please understand that I am not diminishing the impact of breast cancer on your life. But it is best to talk about the issue as matter-of-factly as you would about any other difficult experience in your past. And remember: at least breast cancer, unlike, for example, diabetes, is actually curable.

How do you decide when, in the setting of a dating situation, is best to discuss the changes that breast surgery might have caused in your body? Many women feel that by clearing the air early on, in the conversational stages, you will be able to relax and enjoy the moment if or when the relationship progress to intimacy.

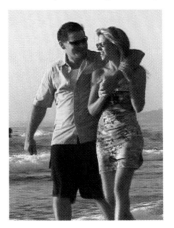

As with so many other aspects of the breast cancer experience, you will find that joining a support group consisting of women who are grappling with the same issues, will do wonders for your confidence.

BEING A YOUNG SURVIVOR

Breast cancer is not unique to "older" women. Today there are over a quarter million women living with breast cancer who are under forty. Being a young breast cancer patient presents a number of unique challenges. You are in a different "place" in your life. You might be looking for a date, rather than celebrating a thirtieth wedding anniversary. You may be fresh out of school, instead of planning your retirement party. You may be looking at five decades of life in front of you, not behind you.

It is particularly important for a young woman to insist that her healthcare providers understand her particular needs. Fertility issues may need to be considered in making a treatment choice. Support groups must be age specific. More attention may be given to retaining appearance and regaining sexuality.

If you are young, take solace in your strengths. Your body can heal faster. You can tolerate chemo better. And you may be more resilient and adaptable than someone who has been set in her ways for the past six decades.

As a breast cancer "minority", a young woman would benefit immensely from interacting with other cancer survivors in her own age bracket. You may want to contact the Young Survival Coalition listed in the Resource section to get you started.

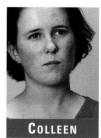

COLLEEN

That is one of the problems of being young with breast cancer. The first support group, everyone was my mom's age. They're talking retirement, you are talking dating. Then my nurse helped me find a younger group, where I could really relate.

New Beginnings

New Perspective

The breast cancer experience can be a powerful incentive to reorder priorities and see life from a different angle. To make a point of finding something enjoyable in every day, in every task. A reminder to stop and smell the roses.

Breast cancer can also be a liberating experience. You may decide to do something you always wanted to do—write poetry, travel, or spend more time with your children.

Healthy Habits

This may be a good time to adopt healthy habits.

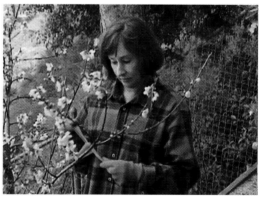

Good Nutrition

Good nutrition may speed your healing after surgery and help you during chemotherapy. Later on, balanced diet, with proper amounts of protein, fats, carbohydrates, and vitamins will help you feel younger and stay healthier. Currently, there is no evidence that breast cancer can be prevented by a low fat or any other type of diet, although certain diets may affect the incidence of other cancers, such as colon cancer.

Physical Activity

You may have done arm exercises as part of your post-surgical recovery. Physical activity will strengthen and energize you, so don't neglect the rest of

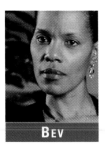

BEV

My old friends are having babies. My new friends are having chemo. I just have to put my energy into dealing with this.

your body. A regular exercise program will help you stay stronger and feel younger. There is also evidence that moderate physical exercise can improve the work of the immune system.

Lifestyle Changes

As a breast cancer survivor you may be at an increased risk for other types of cancer, such as ovarian cancer, lung cancer, or skin cancer. This may be an excellent reason to stop smoking and to take better protective measures when you expose your skin to the sun.

Other lifestyle changes, such as relaxation or meditation, may help you in your personal and professional life as well.

GETTING INVOLVED

As you regain your physical and emotional strength, consider the needs of

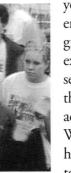

your fellow breast cancer survivors who may be in earlier, or in more difficult stages of their recovery, and could greatly benefit from someone to guide them through the experience. Many organizations listed in the Resources section need volunteers who can help other women in their struggle with breast cancer. Whether as a patient advocate who helps mold breast cancer related policy in Washington, a moderator in a local support group, or a helping hand for a friend, you will find that contributing to the cause is an enriching and uplifting experience.

Race for the Cure by Susan G. Komen Foundation

RECOMMENDATIONS FOR YOUR FAMILY MEMBERS

Although the majority of cases of breast cancer are not hereditary, having a first degree relative, either on the mother's or father's side, does increase the likelihood of developing breast cancer. A good word of advice is to inform your family members of your diagnosis, and suggest that your daughters or sisters be particularly thorough in practicing early detection.

The current recommendations include yearly mammograms starting either at age forty, or at an age that is ten years younger than yours at the time of your diagnosis, whichever is earlier.

For younger women, whose breasts are more dense, and more difficult to be examined by mammography, there are techniques available such as ultrasound and MRI that will help spot smaller changes.

Mammography itself is constantly undergoing refinement. For example, new digital systems make image management easier. There are also computerized programs that enhance the physicians' ability to interpret images rapidly and effectively. And for those women who avoid mammograms for fear of the discomfort caused by the compression, new user-friendly foam pads make much of the discomfort obsolete.

In addition, BSE is important for younger women, who are not yet at the mammogram screening age of over 40. For these women, the only tools readily available are clinical breast examinations and monthly self-examination.

Genetic Testing

One of the questions that women who have been diagnosed with breast cancer ask is, "Should my close relatives be tested for breast cancer genes?" This is not a simple question.

The tests that are available today look for abnormalities in the BRCA genes. If abnormalities are found, then the person has a higher risk of developing breast cancer.

The issue is, what will that person do with the information? At present, the options include prophylactic mastectomy—removal of both breasts as a preemptive measure, or hormone treatment (such as with tamoxifen) that will induce menopause. Neither is an attractive choice. In addition, if the test is negative, it does not mean that the person will not develop breast cancer. If the test is positive, there may be a risk that a health insurance company, or a potential employer will somehow access the information, and use it in a prejudicial way.

The complicated decision of whether to undergo genetic testing should be made with the help of a genetic counselor trained in risk assessment, and the woman must be very clear about the expected benefits and risks.

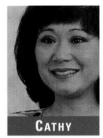

CATHY

One of the most wonderful things about my life after breast cancer is that I've spent a lot of time helping other people. I think breast cancer is a remarkable disease because so many women who are survivors come through that experience and say, "I want to do something to help other people through this."

CHAPTER 14

A Guide for Your Partner

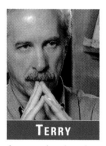

TERRY

I remember hearing a lot from doctors that there wasn't an awful lot you can do, other than hope. I think this is the time when you need to set a direction in terms of your attitude, and building the strength to say, "I'm going to fight this and learn to do what I have to do."

If you had a chance to check the back cover of this book, you probably read that I am a husband of a woman who was diagnosed with breast cancer seventeen years ago, and is very much alive and healthy today. Some of the advice I offer in the next few pages is based on that personal experience. The memory of what I went through is as vivid today as it was back then.

As the partner of a woman with breast cancer, you're probably in as much pain and turmoil as she is. The coming days and months will be challenging. You'll have to deal with your own feelings, as well as give the woman you love the support she needs. A positive attitude will help both of you get through the ordeal.

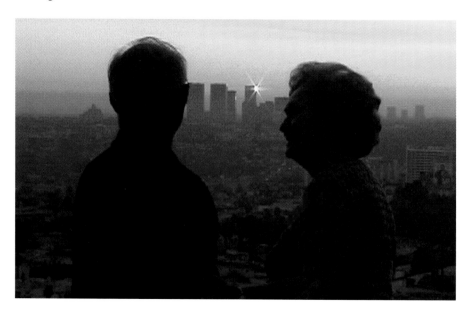

If you can step outside the "cancer" mindset, you will see that this is an opportunity for you and the woman you love to have one of the most rewarding experiences in your life.

WHAT IS BREAST CANCER?

You may know breast cancer as something that requires a big operation and leaves the woman disfigured, or something that is treated with chemotherapy, causing hair to fall out. And something that women usually die of.

In reality, breast cancer that is diagnosed early is one of the most treatable diseases. There has been enormous progress in breast cancer management in the past twenty years. There are effective combinations of treatments that can kill cancer cells, and surgical techniques that give cosmetically pleasing results. In this situation that probably appears pretty dismal to you right now, there are plenty of reasons to be positive.

In the next days or weeks, you should review the appropriate chapters of this book with your partner, and learn with her. Understanding breast cancer and its treatment will help you regain a feeling of control over your life, and will make you a much more effective supporter for the woman you love.

UNDERSTANDING YOUR FEELINGS

"The doctor told me I have breast cancer." These may be the most painful words you'll ever hear from someone you love. Words that bring a flood of emotions—shock, disbelief, confusion—and the inevitable question, "Is she going to die?"

Dealing with these issues is a lot to handle. On top of this, you have an even bigger task. You have to quickly come to grips with your own emotions, so that you can become the main source of support for the woman you love. In the coming days and weeks, you may be asked to play a variety of roles— take notes during medical visits, drive her to chemotherapy sessions, listen without judging, or hold her close when she needs it.

You may feel overcome by the feeling that somehow you must make it all better, and be frustrated when you find out you can't. There is no easy

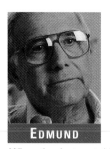

EDMUND

When the doctors told us that Joan had cancer, my first thought was "Is she able to survive this emotionally?" And it did not ever enter my mind that I was going to lose Joan, because we knew that she was positive in her thinking and I was positive in my thinking. And all it was is just a bug that had to be removed.

answer, and no shortcut. Accept what you are feeling. Don't be embarrassed. You are facing a serious problem, and it is normal to feel scared, confused, and weak.

Breast cancer will stress your relationship in countless ways. Your lifestyle will be disrupted—by treatment schedules, or by the new financial burdens that prevent you and your loved one from enjoying your usual activities. The roles each of you played in the relationship may change, and you may find that you are now responsible for tasks that are new to you, or that you are unwilling to tackle. You may have to deal with the side effects of her treatment, such as fatigue, vomiting, or loss of sexual drive. And there will be the turmoil of having to make important decisions while facing the uncertainties of the future.

Fear, anxiety, and sadness will affect how the two of you communicate. Acknowledge these feelings. You can be strong and supportive without holding everything inside. In fact, sharing your feelings honestly with her is the best thing you can do. You may be surprised to find that your loved one appreciates the fact that you can express emotions to her. This sharing improves communication and strengthens your relationship—now, and for the long future.

During the first weeks after her diagnosis you will probably feel like you are riding an emotional roller coaster. There will be days when, after a conversation with your loved one, or a visit to the physician, everything will seem under control, and you will feel strong and optimistic. But that very night, negative thoughts will begin to creep into your head, and you'll feel like all is lost, and there is no hope. You may spend the night pacing, or crying, or wondering what you'll do if you lose the woman you love. By morning you'll remember that there are excellent treatment options, and that her outlook for a healthy life is much better than it seemed a few hours ago. And the world will seem much less gloomy.

These swings of feelings are painful and exhausting, but they are normal. The good news is that with time these emotional tidal waves get smaller and smaller—until they are just ripples in a pond, and you find that you can deal with them.

WHAT DO I DO NOW?

If you are like most men, you will probably be eager to put the emotional issues aside, and spring into "action." "OK, so what do I do now?" is probably high on your list of questions. "How do I solve this problem?"

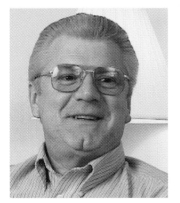

The good news is that you are in a position to contribute greatly to the peace of mind and success of treatment for your loved one. As the husband, partner, "significant other" or principal caregiver, you are in the best position to influence the attitude with which she accepts her diagnosis. And that can make all the difference!

Be as thoughtful as you can in your words and actions. What you do and say in the first few minutes and days after she hears her diagnosis, will make a great difference in how she feels about it herself. Your reaction will play an important role in her physical and mental recovery, so try to be as positive and supportive as you can. One of the most constructive steps you can take is to get involved in her care from the very beginning.

Learn all you can about the disease and the most current treatment options. Search the net, read books, ask questions. Take the time to discuss the information that the two of you gathered, and compare your impressions. Help her stay focused and not go off on tangents.

Accompany her on visits to her healthcare specialists. Bring a list of questions you want answered. Take notes, or use a tape recorder, so you can review the information you received. Don't be disappointed by how little you understand at first. First of all, you are listening through a thick curtain of emotional turmoil. Second, breast cancer treatment is a complex topic, and no one can be expected to grasp all the details on the first pass. Trust me on this. I am a doctor, and I understood next to nothing during the first few visits. If nothing else, your mere presence will provide emotional support and a second set of ears.

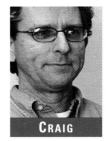

CRAIG

I think that the most useful thing a spouse can do for a woman who has just found out she has cancer is assure her that you're not going to walk away and leave her.

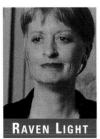

RAVEN LIGHT

Once I was diagnosed, I kind of expected that my lover would just go her way, but she didn't at all. She stayed with me the whole time. From her I learned unconditional love for the first time in my life.

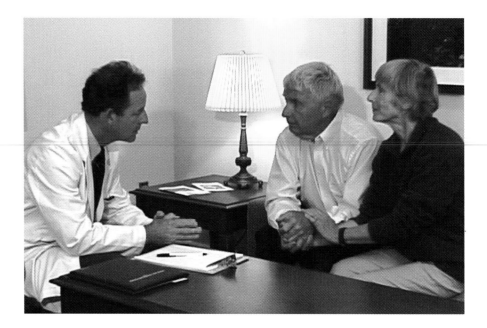

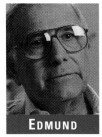

EDMUND

Help your spouse not to dwell on the bad features. Be positive. Look forward to what tomorrow brings, because tomorrow will be a better day than today. Enjoy getting old together.

If you or your partner feel you need a second opinion, don't hesitate to ask her physician for a referral, or seek one on your own. For something as important as breast cancer treatment, you owe it to yourselves to leave no avenue unexplored. Some of the decisions you two will be making are not reversible, so now is the time to really scrutinize your plan. Don't be afraid to "offend" her physician by asking for a referral to someone else. No reputable healthcare professional will resent your request.

Bear in mind that the diagnosis of breast cancer is almost never an emergency. The few exceptions include inflammatory breast cancer that tends to be rapidly growing and should be treated as soon as possible. In most other cases, you and your partner have several weeks to research your options, and make important treatment decisions. Do not let anyone or anything rush you.

Here is the part that you might find to be the most difficult: you must remember that the final decisions about treatment will be hers. Being supportive and helpful does not mean taking over. If you have been in this relationship for some time, you hopefully have learned when to argue, when to persuade, and when to just step back and say, "Honey, if that is what you want to do, I am there for you one hundred percent."

What She Needs From You

Emotional Support

Along with the fear of losing her femininity, and possibly her life, what a woman fears most at this time is that you, the one she loves, will abandon her. Emotional support is perhaps the single most important item you can contribute. Knowing that you will be there for her, no matter what, and that you still find her lovable, desirable, and attractive will help her face her diagnosis and tolerate her treatments better than anything else.

You can also help by creating a safe place for her to express her emotions. This means allowing her to grieve in her own way, without making judgments about the "appropriateness" of her behavior.

If you find verbal communication difficult, and choose to hide in your job or in an outside activity, she may perceive this behavior as a withdrawal of your love. Her well being, and the survival of your relationship itself, depends on your willingness to communicate openly. You don't need to make long speeches. Holding her hand, sitting close to her, putting an arm around her, will communicate how much she means to you in ways words can't express.

Most people, especially men, are upset by tearful outbursts, so your first reaction to her crying may be an attempt to "fix it" or somehow "make it all better." But remember that tears are a healthy response. You and she know that there is no easy fix, and to pretend otherwise only delays the grieving that must take place before healing begins.

Anger is also a normal response. Breast cancer is no one's fault, but anger needs an outlet. She may lash out at the closest person during such times. That might be you. The important thing to remember is that despite what she says, she is not angry at you, but at her loss of control over her life. This stage will pass, and she needs to know you'll still be there for her. Help direct that anger into action, to fight against the cancer and depression.

Some women withdraw and refuse to share their feelings, rejecting your efforts at being close. This may be the most difficult reaction to deal with, and may require outside help to reestablish open communications.

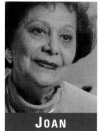

JOAN

There isn't anything that we didn't share. Every word, every feeling, every little thing that went on, we shared. I don't think I could have gone through it without him. He has never said anything that hasn't been, "You're beautiful." And he wasn't afraid to look at the scar and say, "Oh, look how much improvement, isn't that great?" He made me feel wonderful. He made me feel like a star.

SIGNS THAT MAY INDICATE CLINICAL DEPRESSION

- Ongoing sadness and negative statements ("I'm not worth anything anymore." "I hate my life.") lasting a period of weeks rather than days.

- Withdrawing from all normal activities or social/family interactions.

- Physical complaints: sleeplessness or sleeping too much, continual tiredness, over- or under-eating that last a long time.

If your partner displays any of these patterns consistently for two or three weeks, notify her doctor.

Some degree of depression is also to be expected. How do you know if your partner's mood is normal, or if she has a severe depression that requires treatment? This is an important question, because depression can adversely affect her treatment.

It is normal to have short periods of sadness, "blue moods", apathy, or loss of interest in daily activities. You can help her overcome these feelings on your own. But a more serious form of depression, called clinical depression, with prolonged feelings of sadness and loss of interest in all activities, can adversely affect her treatment, and should be managed by a professional.

Once chemotherapy or radiation treatment is completed, your partner may be overcome with feelings of panic or powerlessness that come from the perception that she is no longer being actively treated. It is important to acknowledge these feelings, then focus on the positive aspects of completing the treatment. There is scientific evidence that a positive mind-set can lead to an improved outcome. A supportive and upbeat attitude on your part will be contagious, and is one of the best ways to help her through the weeks or months of treatment.

A few simple techniques that will improve communications

- Make opening statements that let your partner know you're willing to listen. Comments like, "How do you feel about..." let her know that it's okay to open up on an emotional level.
- Reassure her that she has been truly understood by repeating what you heard in your own words.
- Use nonverbal (body language) techniques to convey how you feel about her. Hand holding, and looking directly at her when she speaks tell her that your love and concern are real.
- Avoid judgmental comments like, "You shouldn't..." or, "Don't say that." Such statements block true communication by minimizing or invalidating the other person's feelings.
- Be careful with comments like, "Don't worry," or, "Nothing will happen." Having a positive attitude doesn't mean being unrealistic.

Reassurance About Her Appearance

An unreconstructed mastectomy, or baldness caused by chemotherapy will result in dramatic changes in appearance that will often make the woman feel that her partner will no longer find her attractive. A woman's acceptance of her changed body often depends on your reaction to it. You need to prepare yourself accordingly.

Looking at the mastectomy scar or at the reconstructed breast for the first time can be very frightening. Aside from the change in the familiar look of your loved one, there is the shock of seeing injured skin, perhaps bloody bandages, and drain bulbs full of drainage fluid. If you are at all sensitive to this, it may be a little shocking. But try to keep in mind that once it is healed, the scar will look infinitely better. The swelling, bruising, ß and bandages will be replaced by a clean white line. Try to be as sensitive and accepting as you can. Give her the type of response that you'd like to hear if you were in a similar situation.

Some women have no trouble looking at the surgical site together with their partners at the earliest opportunity. Others choose to view the scar gradually, sometimes alone, or in subdued lighting, or under the cover of an attractive nightgown. Respect her wishes, and be positive and reassuring when you look at her. What is important is not how her chest looks, but the fact that she is still the same woman you love.

Sexual Intimacy

When is the right time for resuming sexual relations? There is nothing about breast cancer that would prevent intimate contact, even if the dressings and drains are still in place. The deciding factor is your partner's, and your, readiness.

Surgery can be exhausting and debilitating. Tenderness around the surgical site, or loss of sensation in the nipple can interfere with physical pleasure. Wearing a natural-looking prosthesis, or having her partner touch other areas of her body, can help a woman refocus sensation and regain interest in intimacy.

Preoccupation with the cancer and its treatment will probably decrease your and her interest in sexual intimacy. Chemotherapy, in particular, can sap the energy and the motivation out of any sexual relations.

QUESTIONS TO ASK HER DOCTOR:

☐ Will there be loss of sensation in the breast area?

☐ Will chemotherapy cause her hair to fall out?

☐ Can we see pictures of what the surgical scar could look like?

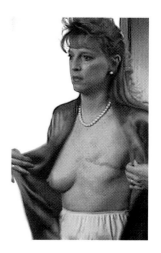

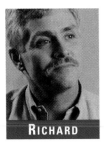

RICHARD

I was intrigued by the fact that Carol had one breast that was quite different than the other. But as far as being shocked, or afraid to touch, not at all. That part did not bother me. It was just, "Ok, this is Carol. This is part of the package. I like the package."

When the time is right, there are a number of small things you can do to rekindle her sexual interest. Make a date with her, give her a foot rub, take a shower together, watch an erotic movie. Try new positions that may be more comfortable. But be patient and know that for many months, perhaps even a year, your sexual interaction may not be the same as it was before.

Help with Daily Activities

After she comes home from the hospital, your partner will have days of physical and emotional exhaustion, and will need your help to handle even the most mundane daily activities. Some women need more help than others. The hard part may be determining how much help she wants. Ask her what she feels like doing on a given day. Look for physical signs of how tired she might be, but avoid "babying" her. Too much help may be as inappropriate as too little. The goal is to return to as normal a life as possible without causing either of you excess stress.

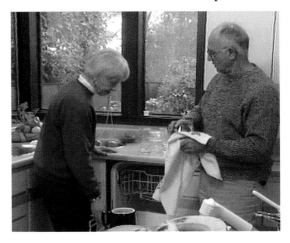

In the early stages of her treatment she may be overcome with a barrage of well-wishing friends and relatives. At first you might feel elated by this, but soon you will find that there is such a thing as too much help and sympathy. You will need to act as the gate keeper—"well-wisher wrangler" as I called my role. Alternately, you can appoint a specific person to channel all the good will coming at the two of you.

To avoid alienating friends and relatives, you might want to delegate specific tasks to various people, such as walking the dog, shopping for groceries, driving the car pool, keeping other friends informed, and so on. That way, everyone feels involved, and the necessities of life are attended to.

If you have children at home, they will need the time and support your partner may not always be able to give them. One of the most helpful things you can provide is a special time or activity that all family members can participate in—for example, renting a movie or going on a picnic.

You also may be required to deal with financial or insurance issues. There are some things you can do to make an unpleasant task much easier:

- Contact your insurance company at the time of diagnosis to find out their policies on hospital admissions, additional medical opinions, filing of claims and billing, etc.
- Keep a written record of your contacts with insurance company representatives, including names, dates, and times.
- Write down appointment dates and doctors' names. Get a copy of all billing forms, which should include procedures, medications, and supplies used.
- Keep all bills, charges, and related forms together in one place for easy retrieval later.
- Don't forget to keep up insurance premiums. You'll be glad you remembered this critical step later.

MEETING YOUR OWN NEEDS

Finding Support for You

The combination of emotional stress, your regular work, and added activities around the home can take a toll on you. You can't afford to exhaust yourself physically or emotionally. No matter how well you think you are handling the situation, you will benefit both you and the woman you love by finding a support person for yourself. A friend, another family member, a religious leader, or a professional counselor who can help you verbalize any feelings and thoughts that you don't want to share with your partner at this particular time.

This support person will help you sort it all out, and work on a plan of action. Talking to other partners of women with breast cancer and participating in support groups can also give you concrete ideas on how to cope. Seeking this form of support for you is not a sign of weakness, but of your wisdom.

SUGGESTIONS FOR FRIENDS WHO WANT TO HELP

- Stop by and bring a newspaper
- Bring the mail or other materials from the office
- Help redecorate a room
- Organize a getaway weekend for both of you
- Drop by and watch a favorite TV program
- Drive her to a chemotherapy session
- Invite the whole family out for a meal

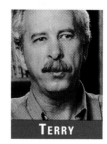

TERRY

It's hard to go and talk to the guys at the office about your wife's mastectomy. I mean, guys just don't open up that much and so there were things that I didn't have anybody to really talk to about. It would have been helpful to have had some support element, whatever it might be.

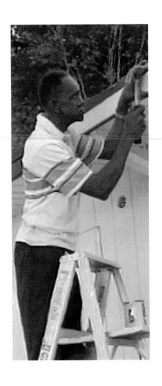

Dealing with the Workload

As the primary support person, you will have a major role in keeping up with your family's daily activities during a difficult time. There will be times when you may feel overwhelmed by the entire burden. Before that occurs, sit down with your partner and make plans:

• Make a list of tasks that need to be done on a daily basis (food preparation, child care). Try to concentrate on activities that really are essential, and put off the unnecessary niceties.

• As people contact you and ask "How can I help?" give them specific tasks that will be truly helpful for you and your partner.

• If you have the financial means, you may want to hire help. Even having someone a few hours a week can ease the situation.

• If you have children, get them more involved in the daily activities. Even young children can be given simple tasks to do around the house, like picking up their toys or setting the dinner table. Actively participating in daily activities gives them a way to cope with their own fears.

MY PERSONAL EXPERIENCE AS THE PARTNER OF A WOMAN WITH BREAST CANCER

Seventeen years ago, at the age of 43, my wife went for what we thought would be a routine mammogram of a lump I found in her breast five days earlier. Just as I was starting to realize that she had been gone too long, the radiologist called. "Dr. Lange, we are looking at your wife's mammograms. It looks like she has a malig-

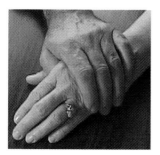

nancy." Just like that. The message was particularly devastating because there wasn't that moment of confusion, that buffer of uncertainty to soften the blow of what I had just heard.

I knew what "malignant" meant. Cancer, mastectomy, chemotherapy, death. I stopped thinking, got in my car, and went down to the radiology facility to pick up my wife.

The most important contribution—sometimes I think it was the only contribution—I made to my wife's recovery, was the attitude I took toward her illness. The thought of being left alone to raise two young children, without the woman I loved, was too frightening a prospect. So I simply decided she was not going to die, and that was that. It was not an option. It was not acceptable. It was my will against the disease, and I was determined to win the battle. In retrospect, we both feel that somehow that mind-set, however irrational, made the difference in her being a survivor.

Another, perhaps equally significant form of support was my wholehearted, unequivocal, and immediate assurance to her that I absolutely did not care what form of surgery she may need, and would love her and find her attractive no matter how she looked. Even today, so many years later, she says that it was this attitude that helped her retain her self-image.

In terms of logistical support, "relative wrangling" was definitely a challenge. Both of us come from European families, with their characteristic exaggerated (often grossly exaggerated) response to a diagnosis of cancer. "Oh, my God, how terrible, the poor thing... (read: *she is going to die*). What are you going to do?" To avoid the negative feelings such outbursts would generate, I decided to paint a much rosier picture of her prognosis, and insisted that no one treat her as a sick person.

CHAPTER 15

Advanced Breast Cancer

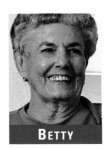

BETTY

It is hard to deal with it the first time. The second time is even harder, but at least you have a better understanding of what to expect. Good thing I didn't throw the wig away.

If you were diagnosed with early-stage breast cancer—in other words, if your tumor has not spread to other parts of your body (Stages 0-III) then the information that you need is contained in other chapters. You may safely skip this chapter, which deals with advanced breast cancer.

What is advanced breast cancer? Advanced, or metastatic, breast cancer is cancer that has spread beyond the breast and past the lymph nodes, to form metastases in other parts of the body, such lungs, liver, brain, and bones. This stage is called Stage IV cancer. About one in ten breast cancers are Stage IV when they are first diagnosed.

Advanced breast cancer may also be a cancer that "came back." In this case, it is also called recurrent cancer.

RECURRENT BREAST CANCER

Sometimes, after the initial treatment, your physician may find evidence that the cancer "came back"?in other words, that you have a recurrence. The recurrence may be local (a small lesion in the breast, along the incision, or near the chest wall), regional (in and around the lymph nodes), or it may be in the form of distant metastases in remote organs of the body. Cancer recurrences usually occur within two to six years after the initial diagnosis, but sometimes even decades later.

You will undergo additional testing to make sure that there are no cancer sites elsewhere in your body. The tests are probably already familiar to you from your first encounter with breast cancer. They include MRI, CT, bone scans, and other means of pinpointing areas where cancer may have spread—locally or to distant areas. At that time the decision will be made regarding additional treatment.

A local recurrence will generally be treated with the same approach as an original cancer: surgery, with or without radiation therapy, and possibly chemotherapy or hormone therapy, depending on the size of the tumor and cell grade.

In advanced stages, breast cancer spreads to the lungs, liver, brain, bones and soft tissues. If the recurrence is in another part of the body, rather than in the breast area, treatment will require a systemic approach targeting the entire body. Recurrences that are found in other organs have a much more serious impact on the course of your disease than local recurrences such as may be found near the lumpectomy scar.

TREATMENT OF ADVANCED/METASTATIC BREAST CANCER

Sometimes, despite the best efforts for early detection, the cancer is not found until it is Stage IV --it has spread to other parts of the body. The reality of Stage IV cancer (advanced breast cancer and recurrent breast cancer with regional and distant metastases) is that it is usually not possible to remove this cancer completely from your body. Most treatments for advanced/metastatic breast cancer will try to shrink the tumor or to stop it from growing. The good news is that today there are many treatment methods that can greatly improve your quality of life, and extend the time that you remain free of any evidence of the disease.

Surgery

Surgery in the form of a lumpectomy or mastectomy is the key treatment in early breast cancer. But it is not as useful in advanced breast cancer, that presents with metastases outside the breast. If you were diagnosed with a breast cancer that is present in your breast and in other parts of your body, it is possible that your healthcare team may suggest that you forego a mastectomy. The reason is that the greatest threat to your health comes not from the tumor in the breast, but from the distant metastases that damage other organs, which generally are difficult to treat surgically.

Surgery may play a role in removing a small, solitary tumor from your lung

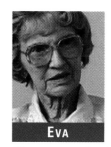

EVA

After you cry and rant and rave, then at some point you go, "OK, this isn't going away." And then you can channel your energy into making the very best you can of the situation.

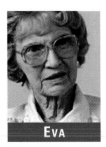

EVA

At first Mike and I threw ourselves into the search for a cure. Something had to exist, something western medicine overlooked. Some secret potion? After a while we realized we were just running away from reality.

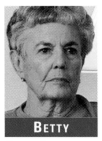

BETTY

Remember, at some point docs will only tell you what you ask. So ask. Don't imagine horrors. The truth may not be as harsh as your imagination.

or liver, or another part of the body where it is applying pressure on another organ. This is called palliative surgery.

Radiation Therapy

Radiation therapy may be used to shrink metastases in distant organs. The treatment will be done by external beam rather than by brachytherapy (see Chapter 6). You may need only a few treatments, rather than the entire five to seven week course.

Chemotherapy, Hormone Therapy and Immunotherapy

In early cancer, chemotherapy is given to destroy undetectable cells that may or may not have spread through the body, and there is no way to monitor the success of the therapy.

In advanced cancer, if your healthcare team may be able to use X-rays or CT scans to observe the tumor as it shrinks from the chemotherapy. If progress is unsatisfactory, the physician will be able to switch to another drug, or a combination of drugs. You may want to review Chapter 7 for tips on how to deal with side effects of chemotherapy.

Bones are common first sites to which breast cancer tends to spread. You may be treated with additional drugs called bisphosphonates that specifically target bone metastases, and are given with your regular chemotherapy or hormone therapy.

Hormone therapy as well as immunotherapy can also be used effectively to control the growth and spread of advanced breast cancer. The principles are described in Chapter 8.

A new direction in chemotherapy is oral chemotherapy. One such agent, a form of 5-FU is called Xeloda. It is taken as a twice-daily pill at home, rather than by injection into a vein at the chemotherapy facility a time-saving and discomfort-reducing feature that many women appreciate. The drug has a unique activation mechanism that makes it active mostly within tumor cells, which reduces the side-effects. So women taking Xeloda have minimal hair loss, and their blood producing bone marrow is affected little, if at all, minimizing their chances of infections. As with any self-adminis-

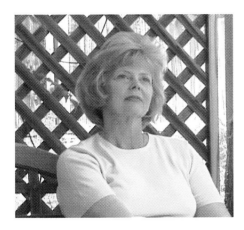

tered therapy, Xeloda does require that the patient and her caregiver be particularly attentive to proper dosages, timing, and any side effects.

COPING WITH ADVANCED BREAST CANCER

It is important for you and your healthcare professionals to be realistic about the probable course of advanced breast cancer. But it is just as important for you to remember that every woman is different, and every cancer runs a different course. Your task now is to avail yourself of all possible resources, and become determined to work toward the best outcome possible.

There are many excellent organizations listed in the Resource section that will help guide you on your quest for information. In addition, you may seek out one of several superb books written by women who "have been there before" and offer their unique insights into dealing with this challenging issue.

Resources

On the following pages you'll find an extensive list of groups, organizations, and businesses that can help you in your fight against breast cancer. They are divided into categories of general resources, sources of help with appearance, and professional organizations.

GENERAL RESOURCES

The American Cancer Society

National Office:
1599 Clifton Road NE
Atlanta, GA 30329
404-320-3333 or 800-ACS-2345
Website: www.cancer.org

The American Cancer Society (ACS) is the nationwide community-based volunteer health organization dedicated to eliminating cancer as a major health problem. Free booklets, videos, and other materials are available from your local chapter or by calling 800-ACS-2345.

ACS also operates the *Reach to Recovery* program which can match you with a volunteer who has had the same kind of treatment you are considering. *The Look Good...Feel Better* program helps women deal with changes in their appearance caused by cancer treatment.

The Australian Cancer Society

70 William Street
East Sydney NSW 2011, Australia
02 9380 9022
Website: www.cancer.org.au

An Australian organization similar to the American Cancer Society.

Australian New Zealand Breast Cancer Clinical Trials Group

Department of Clinical Oncology
Newcastle Mater Hospital
Waratah NSW 2298, Australia
+61 2 4921 1155

A group dedicated to the research of breast cancer in Austalia and New Zealand. Contact them for more information on the latest clinical trials being conducted.

Breastcancer.org

111 Forest Avenue IR
Narberth, PA 19072
Website: www.breastcancer.org

Non-profit organization dedicated to providing accurate and current online information about breast cancer.

Breast Cancer Care

Kiln House, 210 New Kings Road
London SW6 4NZ
0207-384-2984 (United Kingdom)

Breast Cancer Care is an organization in the United Kingdom that offers free information, help and support to those affected by breast cancer. Their services include a volunteer service, national help-line, prosthesis fitting, and a wide range of information, from booklets to audio tapes.

Breast Cancer Early Detection Program /
Breast & Cervical Cancer Control Program;
California Department of Health Services

P.O. Box 942732, MS-294
Sacramento, CA 94234-7320
800-511-2300

The California Department of Health Services and the Center for Disease Control and Prevention fund programs which provide free clinical breast examinations and mammograms to low-income, uninsured, or underinsured women. Services are available to women 40 and older. Free pap smears are offered to women 25 and older. The California program also covers diagnostics.

Women in California can call the toll-free number to find out if they qualify and to get referrals to participating providers in their area. For programs outside California, contact your state health department and ask for the Breast and Cervical Cancer Program.

Breast Cancer Resource Committee /
A Beacon of Hope

2005 Belmont Street, NW
Washington, DC 20009
202-463-8040
Website: www.afamerica.com

Conducts local and national breast cancer educational programs targeting African-American women and other minorities who have limited access to breast-care treatment.

California Breast Cancer Organizations

254 East Grand Street, Ste. 205
Escondido, CA 92025
760-839-1491

A coalition of breast cancer organizations throughout California, educating, empowering and advocating for California women.

Camp Healthcare
P.O. Box 89
Jackson, MI 49204
800-492-1088
Website: www.camphealthcare.com

Offers products for women who have had surgery for breast cancer. These products include bras, breast forms, swimwear, and accessories for the postmastectomy woman.

Canadian Breast Cancer Foundation
790 Bay Street, Suite 1000
Toronto, Ontario M5G 1N8, Canada
800-387-9816 or 416-596-6773

This organization offers financial support for research and treatment of breast cancer, encourages and coordinates training, public information and all related resources.

Canadian Cancer Society

National Office
10 Alcorn Avenue, Suite 200
Toronto, Ontario
M4V 3B1
416-961-7223
Website: www.cancer.ca

A national community-based organization of volunteers, whose mission is the eradication of cancer and the enhancement of the quality of life of people living with cancer. They provide peer support, cancer information, summer camps, and financial-aid information.

Cancer Care Inc.

275 Seventh Avenue
New York, NY 10001
212-712-8080: For a Cancer Care social worker.
800-813-4673: Toll-free counseling line.
Website: www.cancercare.org
E-Mail: info@cancercare.org

A social service agency that helps patients and their families cope with the impact of cancer. Services include professional counseling, financial assistance, information and referral, and insurance counseling, at no cost to the client. Direct services are limited to the greater New York metropolitan area, but callers will be referred to similar assistance available in their areas. Services are also provided in Spanish.

CancerBACUP

3 Bath Place, Rivington Street
London EC2A 3JR, United Kingdom
Information: 0808 800 1234, or 020 7613 2121
Website: www.cancerbacup.org.uk

CancerBACUP is a leading national charity in the U.K. providing information, counseling and support for people with cancer, their families and friends. It is staffed by specialist cancer nurses and professional counselors. CancerBACUP publishes booklets on specific cancers, treatments and on living wtih cancer.

Cancerfacts.com

Website: www.cancerfacts.com

Provides one-stop online resources to accurate, current and personalized information so that patients can take an active part in the management of their disease and help determine their future.

Cancer Institute

Franklin Square Hospital Center
9000 Franklin Square Drive
Baltimore, MD 21237
443-777-7900
Website: www.franklinsquare.org

Provides services to patients and their families in accessing current cancer treatment information.

Fertile Hope

42 W. 24th Street
New York, NY 10010
888-994-HOPE
Website: www.fertilehope.org

A non-profit dedicated to providing support and educational information to cancer patients dealing with fertility issues, before, during and after treatment.

Gilda's Club Worldwide

195 West Houston Street
New York, NY 10014-4872
212-647-9700
Website: www.gildasclub.org

A free cancer support community for people living
with cancer, their families and friends. Provides social
and emotional support through support groups, lec-
tures, workshops and social events. There are 26 clubs
worldwide.

Institute for Health and Healing Library

2040 Webster Street
San Francisco, CA 94115
415-600-3681 (recorded information) or
415-923-3681 (direct line)

Medical library for the general public. The collection
includes current information from professional medical literature, popular health publications, and alternative therapy resources. Books and tapes are available
for sale through the bookstore catalog.

Kids Konnected

Kids Konnected
27071 Cabot Road, Suite 102
Laguna Hills, CA 92653
Hotline: 800-899-2866 or 949-582-5443
Website: www.kidskonnected.org
E-mail: info@kidskonnected.org

Kids Konnected is a national non-profit that provides
age specific and cancer specific resources and emotional support for kids ages 4-17 who have a parent with
cancer. The monthly peer support groups are run by
kids and led by licensed therapist. Other services that
are provided are: summer camps, Youth Leadership
Training, and grief workshops. .

Living Beyond Breast Cancer

10 E. Athens Avenue, Suite 204
Ardmore, PA 19003
610-645-4567
Website: www.lbbc.org

A national educational non-profit committed to
empowering all women affected by breast cancer to
live as long as possible with the best quality of life.

Men Against Breast Cancer

P.O. Box 150
Adamstown, MD 21710
866-547-6222
Website: www.menagainstbreastcancer.org

National non-profit designed to provide support services to educate and empower men so that they may
be effective caregivers when breast cancer affects their
partners.

Mentor Corporation

5425 Hollister Avenue
Santa Barbara, CA 93111
800-525-0245

Mentor Corporation manufactures a wide variety of
silicone and saline-filled breast prostheses. Several of
these products can be used both as expanders and as
permanent prostheses, enabling a woman to benefit
from a single-stage reconstruction.

Mautner Projects for Lesbians with Cancer

1707 L Street, NW, Suite 500
Washington, DC 20036
202-332-5536
Fax: 202-332-0662
Website: www.mautnerproject.org

Provides support services to lesbians with cancer and their families. Educates lesbians about cancer, and healthcare professionals about working with lesbians.

National Breast Cancer Foundation, Inc.

One Hanover Park
16633 North Dallas Parkway, Suite 600
Addison, TX 75001
Website: www.nationalbreastcancer.org

National non-profit that provides awareness of breast cancer through education and provides free mammograms for those in need.

National Cancer Institute

Cancer Information Service
Office of Cancer Communications
Bethesda, MD 20892
800-4-CANCER (1-800-422-6237)
Hawaii, on Oahu: 808-586-5853
Alaska: 800-638-6070
Website: www.cancernet.nci.nih.gov

The National Cancer Institute (NCI) is part of the National Institutes of Health and is the federal government's principal agency for cancer research and control.

The Cancer Information Service (CIS) of the NCI offers free written materials and information about cancer prevention and control, treatment, support services, medical facilities, second opinion centers, and clinical trials. The hotline is operated by a network of authorized comprehensive cancer centers. Spanish speaking staff members are available. All services are free.

CancerFax, a service of the NCI, provides treatment information summaries from the Physician Data Query (PDQ) for health care professionals and patients; information on supportive care, screening, prevention, and anticancer drugs; as well as fact sheets, news, and bulletins from the NCI. Spanish versions are available. CancerFax can be reached at 800-624-2511.

National Coalition for Cancer Survivorship

NCCS
1010 Wayne Avenue, Suite 770
Silver Spring, MD 20910
301-650-9127
Website: www.canceradvocacy.org

The oldest survivor-led advocacy organization working on behalf of people with cancer. Advocates for quality cancer care for all Americans.

National Family Caregivers Association

10400 Connecticut Avenue, Suite 500
Kensington, MD 20895-3944
800-896-3650
Website: www.nfcacares.org

Provides education and support to patients and their families to improve the overall quality of life of caregiving families and minimizing the disparities between caregivers and patients.

National Lymphedema Network

Latham Square, 1611 Telegraph Avenue, Suite 1111
Oakland, CA 94612-2138
800-541-3259 or 415-921-1306
Website: www.lymphnet.org
E-mail: nln@lymphnet.org

An internationally recognized non-profit organization providing assistance and information to women with lymphedema.

National Women's Health Network

514 10th Street NW, Suite 400
Washington, DC 20004
202-347-1140
202-628-7814 (health information)
Website: www.nwhn@nwhn.org

A public-interest organization devoted only to women and health. Advocacy for legislative issues.

NHMRC National Breast Cancer Centre

92 Parramatta Road
Campertown NSW 1450 Australia
Website: www.nhmrc.gov.au
+61 2 9036-3030

This center, operated by the National Health and Medical Research Council, provides information and resources for women in Australia.

Oncolink

Website: www.oncolink.org

An internet-based resource designed by the University of Pennsylvania Medical Center to collect and disseminate information relevant to the field of oncology to patients, families, and healthcare providers.

People Living with Cancer

1900 Duke Street, Suite 200
Alexandria, VA 22314
703-797-1914
Website: www.peoplelivingwithcancer.org

A patient-information website of the American Society of Clinical Oncology. Provides oncologist-approved information on breast cancer and its treatments, clinical trials, coping and side effects. Services include live chats, drug database, and links to patient-support organizations.

Pregnant with Cancer

P.O. Box 1243
Buffalo, NY 14220
800-743-6724
Website: www.pregnantwithcancer.org

A national support network of women who have been diagnosed with breast cancer during pregnancy. Member-led support, share experiences and offer hope.

Quebec Breast Cancer
Information Exchange Network

Centre hospitalier de l'Université de Montréal,
Hôtel-Dieu Campus
3840 Saint-Urbain Street
Montréal, Quebec   H2W1T8, Canada
Website: phac-aspc.gc.ca

An organization providing information, support and
resources for French speaking women in Canada.

SHARE

1501 Broadway, Suite 704A
New York, NY 10036
Hotlines : 212-382-2111 or 212-719-4454 (Spanish)
Office: 212-719-0364
Website: www.sharecancersupport.org

A non-profit, self-help organization that provides support services for women with breast or ovarian cancer,
and for their families and friends. It offers peer counseling, support groups, hotlines in both English and
Spanish.

Sharsheret

P.O. Box 3245
Teaneck, NJ 07666
866-474-2774
Website: www.sharsheret.org

A national non-profit organization dedicated to
addressing the culturally sensitive issues facing Jewish
women living with breast cancer. Provides links to
peers within the different sectors in the Jewish community who can provide support.

Sisters Network, Inc.

8787 Woodway Drive, Suite 4206
Houston, TX 77063
713-781-0255
Website: www.sistersnetworkinc.org

An African American breast cancer survivorship that
promotes peer support, community awareness, and
education to the African American community.

The Susan G. Komen Breast Cancer Foundation

5005 LBJ Freeway, Suite 250
Dallas, TX 75244
800-I'M-AWARE (800-462-9273)
Website: www.komen.org

Probably the most prestigious and most active breast
cancer advocy organization. Their mission is to eradi-
cate breast cancer as a life-threatening disease by advocating research, education, screening, and treatment.
Komen is the nation's largest private funder of research
dedicated solely to breast cancer. Volunteers work
through chapters and Race for the Cure® events
across the country.

The Wellness Community

919 18th Street, NW
Suite 54
Washington, DC 20006
202-659-9709
Website: www.thewellnesscommunity.org

A national organization dedicated to providing emotional support and education for people with cancer
and their loved ones in a comfortable, home-like setting. Over 22 facilities nationwide. All services are free.

The Women's Cancer Resource Center

5741 Telegraph Avenue
Oakland, CA 94609
510-420-7900
Website: www.wcrc.org

Provides information on breast cancer and health-related issues for women, referrals, educational forums and workshops. The center is well known throughout the lesbian community.

Y-ME National Breast Cancer Organization

212 W. Van Buren Street, Suite 1000
Chicago, IL 60607
Hotline: 800-221-2141 or 800-986-9505 (Spanish)
Website: www.y-me.org
E-mail: help@y-me.org

Y-ME National Breast Cancer Organization ensures, through information, empowerment, and peer support, that no one face breast cancer alone. Its 11 affiliates provide a 24-hour hotline staffed solely by breast cancer survivors. The services include support groups, early-detection workshops, wigs, and prostheses, for women with limited resources. Interpreters are available in 150 languages.

Young Survival Coalition

155 6th Avenue, 10th floor
New York, NY 10013
212-206-6610
Website: www.youngsurvival.org

The only international non-profit network for breast cancer survivors and supporters with a focus on women under 40.

APPEARANCE

Brigher Side Boutique

439 South Cedros Avenue
Solana Beach, CA 92075
800-210-8550 or 858-481-7565

Cancer survivors help other women find breast prostheses, mastectomy bras, swim forms, lingerie and
other post-surgical products.

Look Good ... Feel Better

21 East 40th Street, Suite 1700
New York, NY 10016
212-685-5955
Website: www.lookgoodfeelbetter.org

Organization supported by Cosmetic Executive
Women, Inc., to provide working women with the
resources to continue working through their cancer
treatment.

Nearly Me

626-334-8871 • 800-736-1775

A line of premium-quality breast prostheses, lingerie,
and mastectomy product accessories, including four
styles of silicone gel forms.

Women's Health Boutique

12715 Telge Road
Cypress, TX 77429
888-708-9982
Website: www.w-h-b.com

Eleven national boutiques that offer a variety of innova-
tive health-related merchandise that can also be purchased
discreetly online in the comfort of your own home.

PROFESSIONAL ORGANIZATIONS

American Society of Clinical Oncology
1900 Duke Street, Ste. 200
Alexandria, VA 22314
703-299-0150
Website: www.asco.org

A national medical specialty society representing 21,500 oncologists. The society is a leading cancer organization for scientific and educational exchange and is an active advocate on behalf of cancer patients and their healthcare providers.

American Society of Plastic Surgeons
444 East Algonquin Road
Arlington Heights, IL 60005
1-888-4-PLASTIC
Website: www.plasticsurgery.org

The largest plastic surgery organization in the world; devoted to advancing quality care in plastic surgery. Provides written information on reconstruction, and mails a list of certified plastic surgeons. Visit their website to locate a board-certified surgeon in your area or for additional information about procedures.

Food and Drug Administration (FDA) Information Hotline
5600 Fishers Lane
Rockville, MD 20857
1-888-INFO-FDA (1-888-463-6332)

Provides information regarding breast implants and answers questions about the FDA in general.

National Consortium of Breast Centers (NCBC)
P.O. Box 1334
Warsaw, IN 46581
574-267-8058
Website: www.breastcare.org

Professional membership organization of comprehensive breast centers throughout the nation.

Oncology Nursing Society
501 Holiday Drive
Pittsburgh, PA 15220-2749
Website: www.ons.org

A national organization of more than 30,000 nurses dedicated to patient care, research, education, and administration in the field of oncology. Provides a variety of outstanding educational publications and audio-visual materials.

People Living with Cancer
Offered by American Society of Clinical Oncology
1900 Duke Street, Suite 200
Alexandria, VA 22314
703-299-0150
Website: www.asco.org

This is an extensive patient information website designed to assist patients and families in making informed healthcare decisions. The site provides information on 50 types of cancer, clinical trials, coping, side effects, etc. and helps patients in finding an oncologist and patient support organizations.

Library

BOOKS AND PAMPHLETS

Advanced Breast Cancer
A Guide to Living with Metastatic Disease

Written by Musa Mayer
Edited by Linda Lamb
O'Reilly & Associates, 1998

A few books deal specifically with metastatic cancer, or cancer that has spread beyond the breasts to other parts of the body. Musa Mayer, author of the popular book, *Examing Myself* provides a compassionate approach to the subject.

The Breast Cancer Book of Strength and Courage

Written by Ernie Bodai, M.D.
and Judie Fertig Panneton
Primi Lifestyles, 2002

Uplifting personal stories that offer strength and encouragement to patients and their loved ones.

Breast Cancer: The Complete Guide

Written by Yashar Hirshaut, MD, FACP and Peter I Pressman, MD
Bantam, 2004

An easy-to-follow resource providing up-to-date medical information and practical advice on breast cancer from suspicion of disease through diagnosis, treatment, and follow-up care. An good book written in an easy-to-read, narrative style, filled with examples from the authors' experiences.

Breast Cancer Husband: How to Help your Wife (and Yourself) Through Diagnosis, Treatment and Beyond

Written by Marc Silver
Rodale, 2004
Guidance for partners of women with breast cancer. Provides suggestions on how to support their partners through the cancer journey.

Breast Health: What Every Woman Needs to Know

Written by Vladimir Lange, MD
Brochure - 16 pages
Lange Productions, 2004
888-LANGE-88

This brochure contains valuable information on breast anatomy, benign conditions, early detection, breast cancer, and working with the healthcare provider.

Cancer for Two: An Inspiring True Story and Guide for Cancer Patients and Their Partners

Order from www.ThePatientPartnerProject.org
P.O. Box 824
Twin Peaks, CA 92391
866-725-7877

Book provides the caregivers and the patient with comfort, advice, guidance and understanding of breast cancer and how to support the patient with humor and love.

Confíe en el Mañana: Guia para el tratamiento del cancer de seno

Written by Vladimir Lange, MD
Lange Productions, 1999

The Spanish language version of *Be a Survivor*. This book is not simply a translation; it has been rewritten to reflect the attitudes and needs of Latina women and their families, and features excerpts from interviews with Latina breast cancer survivors.

Dr. Susan Love's Breast Book
Third Edition

Written by Susan M. Love, M.D. with Karen Lindsey
Addison-Wesley Publishing, 2000

A well-known and respected breast surgeon and feminist discusses all conditions of the breast, from benign to malignant. New developments in breast care, screening, diagnosis, treatment options, research, and controversies are clearly presented in a friendly, accessible style. Excellent general reference on all breast health topics.

The Healing Power of Movement: How to Benefit from Physical Activity During Your Cancer Treatment
Written by Lisa Hoffman and with Alison Freeland
Perseus Publishing, 2002

The Healing Power of Movement addresses this significant shift in care recommendations and clearly illustrates fifty specific exercises-from simply sitting up or moving in bed to walking or lifting light weights-for different stages of cancer treatments, and for many different types of cancers.

The Hope Tree: Kids Talk About Breast Cancer

Written by Laura Numeroff, Wendy Schlessel Harpham, David M. McPhail
School & Library Binding, 2001

Drawing on actual accounts, the authors create a fictional support group, which addresses 10 topics familiar to families dealing with the disease.

Ice Bound: A Doctor's Incredible Battle for Survival at the South Pole

Written by Jerri Nielsen
Talk Miramax Books, 2002

This book tells the gripping story of when Dr. Jerri Nielsen made headlines when she discovered a lump in her breast. No flights in or out of Antarctica are possible during the continent's long winter, and Nielsen's account of giving herself chemotherapy is gripping.

"I Flunked my Mammogram!"

Written by Ernie Bodai, MD and Richard Zmuda
B2Z Publishing, 2005

A very concise and user-friendly book on everything a woman needs to know about breast cancer. Dr. Bodai introduced the breast cancer stamp.

Living Beyond Limits

Written by David Spiegel, M.D.
Published by Ballantine Books, 1994

Based on fifteen years of groundbreaking research, Dr. Spiegel outlines a scientifically-proven program to help all people with chronic illnesses enhance the quality of their lives, by taking advantage of the essential healing connection between body and mind.

Living Beyond Breast Cancer

Written by Marissa Weiss, Ellen Weiss
Three Rivers Press, 1998

Written for the over two million women who are living with breast cancer to help them understand the tough issues that they will face as they move beyond treatment.

Living Through Breast Cacner

Written by Carolyn M. Kaelin, Francesca Coltrera
Harvard Medical School, 2005

The author is a breast surgeon and a breast cacner survivor. A helpful book that will inform patients and families who just want the facts.

Medicine and Compassion for Caregivers

Written by Chokvi Nyima Rinpoche
Wisdom Publications, 2004

Helps caregivers become more attentive and compassionate for those that they care for.

Reconstructing Aphrodite

Written by Terry Lorant and Loren Eskenazi, M.D.
Verve Editions, 2002

This book is a unique combination of photographic and surgical artistry, and the courageous stories of women whose lives have been transformed. It also contains detailed information about breast reconstruction and resources to guide someone through the maze of medical decisions that must be made if one's life has been touched by breast cancer.

Taking Time: Support for People With Cancer and the People Who Care About Them

National Cancer Institute, 1996
800-4-CANCER

This book is written as a guide for the patient and her loved ones to help them cope with their fears and deal with their feelings upon being diagnosed with cancer.

Uplift: Secrets from the Sisterhood of Breast Cancer Survivors

Written by Barbara Delinshky
Pocket Books, 2001

This book is an inspiring collection of voices of breast cancer survivors.

Victoria's Secret Catalog Never Stops Coming: And Other Lessons I Learned from Breast Cancer

Written by Jennie Nash
Scribner, 2001

Touching and courageous, this book blends the medical realities of breast cancer with the wise and thoughtful opinions of author Jennie Nash.

Woman to Woman: A Handbook for Women Newly Diagnosed with Breast Cancer

Written by Hester Hill Schnipper LICSW, Joan Feinberg Berns
Wholecare, 1999

Here are compassionate thoughts and advice from survivors aimed at making the first steps on your journey to recovery a positive one.

A Woman's Decision:
Breast Care, Treatment, & Reconstruction
Third Edition

Written by Karen Berger and John Bostwick III, M.D.
Quality Medical Publishing, 1998

A sensitive and authoritative book that will help women assess their options, familiarize themselves with the techniques used in treating cancer, and prepare themselves for what to expect medically and emotionally from reconstructive surgery. Copiously illustrated with outstanding photographs and drawings.

A Woman's Guide to Breast Cancer
Diagnosis and Treatment

California Dept. of Health Services,
Breast Cancer Early Detection Program, 1995
Available from: Breast Cancer Treatment Options,
Medical Board of California
1426 Howe Ave., Suite 54
Sacramento, CA 95825

This booklet is an invaluable guide for the woman who has been diagnosed with breast cancer. A comprehensive overview of all the stages a woman is likely to encounter as she goes from diagnosis to treatment and recovery. Elegant illustrations complement the clearly written and beautifully laid out text. Sidebars summarize information, call out important concepts, and list commonly asked questions. California law mandates that this publication be given to the patient at the time of biopsy, but every woman facing breast cancer should obtain a copy.

VIDEOS AND CD-ROMS

Baby Boomer Be Healthy: Breast Health & Cancer

Video - 23 minutes
Lange Productions, 2001
888-LANGE-88

This program deals with early detection, genetic testing, breast cancer, and treatment options. Other parts of this collection include osteoporosis, continence, estrogen loss, cardiac problems and other conditions affecting women in their 40's and beyond.

Be A Survivor™: Your Interactive Guide
to Breast Cancer Treatment

CD-ROM
Lange Productions, 1999
888-LANGE-88

This multi-award winning CD-ROM, the program on which this book is based, allows you to actually see the procedures and the 3-D animated graphics, and to hear the patient interviews. You can explore the CD-ROM at your own pace, and print lists of resources or questions to ask your healthcare professionals. The program features more than twelve hours of material, including sections on both standard and complementary therapies, breast anatomy, diagnosis and staging, breast cancer resources, help for the patient's life partner, and life after cancer. The CD-ROM, designed for users who are not computer experts, is extremely easy to use: Any topic can be accessed with a simple click of the mouse. On some computers, you can use the program by simply touching the screen with your finger.

Be A Survivor™:
Treatment Options For Breast Cancer

Video - 28 minutes
Lange Productions
888-LANGE-88

This video parallels the content of this book. The program, clearly illustrated with 3-D animated graphics, gives a step-by-step presentation of the treatment process, from needle biopsy to nipple reconstruction. Highlighted with comments from breast cancer survivors, this video is an ideal take-home guide for newly-diagnosed patients and their loved ones.

Breast Facts, The Basics

Video - 8 minutes
Lange Productions, 1998
888-LANGE-88

This videotape provides an excellent introduction to breast health by describing breast anatomy and physiology, breast lumps, "fibrocystic disease," and factors that may contribute to the risk of breast cancer.

B.S.E For Teens—with Jennie Garth Introduction

Video - 7 minutes
Lange Productions, 2002
888-LANGE-88

This program encourages teenagers to learn how breasts look and feel now, when they are healthy, so that they will be more likely to spot a change later on. Beautiful 3-D graphics illustrate anatomy, while an all-teen, multi-ethnic cast clearly demonstrate the latest techniques for breast self examination. Upbeat tempo and an introduction by actress Jennie Garth of Beverly Hills 90210, make this video a hit with teenage audiences. A valuable teaching tool for daughters of women who have been diagnosed with breast cancer.

Companion Video to the Be a Survivor Book

Video - 35 minutes
Lange Productions, 1999
888-LANGE-88.

Women who have "been there" share their stories. The perfect companion to the *Be a Survivor* book, this video brings to life the survivors you've read here with on-screen interviews about their triumphs over breast cancer.

Confie en el Mañana

Video - 40 minutes
Lange Productions
888-LANGE-88

This video is based on the *Be a Survivor™* video. As with the book, the video walks the patient through all stages of the treatment process from inital exams to life after cancer. With excellent graphics and live patient interviews, the newly diagnosed Latina breast cancer patient is given a visual overview of the book.

Focus on Healing

Video - 49 minutes
Enhancement Inc.
Distributed by Lange Productions
888-LANGE-88

"The Lebed Method." This video is a program of exercise specifically designed to meet the needs of breast cancer survivors of all ages and fitness levels. It will help you regain full range of motion, reduce the risk of lymphedema, and improve self image.

The New B.S.E.

Video - 6 minutes
Lange Productions, 2002
888-LANGE-88

This much-acclaimed video follows the latest Susan G. Komen guidelines. Easy to follow demonstrations use 3-D graphics and feature women of a variety of ages and ethnic backgrounds. The program stresses the importance of monthly B.S.E. as part of a breast health routine, and encourages patients to adopt this lifesaving habit. A must for all women, and particularly for close relatives of women diagnosed with breast cancer. Also available in Spanish, Korean, Russian, Ukranian, and Slovak.

Quality Mammography Can Save Your Life

Video - 8 minutes
Lange Productions, 2003
888-LANGE-88

This "must see" video emphasizes that mammography, in combination with breast self examination and clinical examination, can lead to early detection and improve chances of successful treatment. The program outlines the most current recommendations on frequency of mammography—every year for all women, starting at age forty, or starting ten years younger than the age at which a close relative was diagnosed with breast cancer.

Glossary

abscess
A pocket of pus caused by an infection.

AC
Chemotherapy combination of two different drugs: Adriamycin and Cytoxan.

Adriamycin (doxorubicin)
A drug used to kill cancer cells.

Adrucil (5-fluorouracil)
A drug used to kill cancer cells.

anesthesia
Procedure used to make surgery painless, either by local numbing or by putting the patient to sleep. It is usually performed by an anesthesiologist or a nurse anesthetist.

antiemetic
A medicine that relieves nausea (feeling sick to the stomach) and vomiting (throwing up).

antioxidant
Compounds which slow the deterioration (or oxidation) of cells in the body. Vitamins C and E, as well as beta-carotene are antioxidants.

Arimidex (anastrozole)
A drug for treatment of advanced breast cancer in postmenopausal women.

aspiration
Removal of liquid or tissue cells from a cyst or other structure in the breast, by inserting a needle and drawing (aspirating) fluid into a syringe.

bank blood
Blood that has been donated and stored for later use.

bilateral
Something that is present on both sides of the body. For example, a bilateral mastectomy is a surgery where both breasts are removed.

blood cell count
A test that measures the number of red blood cells, white blood cells, and platelets in a blood sample. This test helps evaluate the effect of chemotherapy on the bone marrow where the blood cells are produced.

brachytherapy
A form of radiation therapy in which the source of the radiation is placed close to, or implanted in, the body.

breast form
Something with the shape and texture of a breast, created with tissue or with a prosthetic.

CAF
Chemotherapy combination of three different drugs: Cytoxan, Adriamycin, and 5-fluorouracil.

carbohydrate
A chemical compound which serves as a basic source of energy. Foods high in carbohydrates include sugars and starches such as bread and pasta.

carcinoembryonic antigen (CEA)
Blood test used to follow women with metastatic breast cancer to help determine if the treatments are working.

carcinogen
Any substance that initiates or promotes the development of cancer.

carcinoma
a form of cancer that develops in the lining of the organs of the body, such as the skin, the uterus, the lungs, or the breast.

carcinoma in situ
A carcinoma that has not spread outside the area where it began.

catheter
A tube used to allow fluid to pass into or out of the body.

cell
The basic building block of all organisms. Individual cells can only be seen when they are magnified through a microscope.

chromosome
One of the many strands of DNA material within the cell that carries genetic information.

circulatory system
The system consisting of the heart and blood vessels which provides blood to all parts of the body.

CMF
Chemotherapy combination of three different drugs: Cytoxan, methotrexate, and 5-fluorouracil.

colony stimulating factors
Chemotherapy additives which stimulate the bone marrow. May be required to maintain adequate blood cell counts during chemotherapy treatment.

combination chemotherapy
Use of two or more chemicals to achieve maximum damage to tumor cells.

cyst
A sac-like structure that contains liquid or semi-solid material.

Cytoxan (cyclophosphamide)
A drug used to kill cancer cells.

DCIS
Abbreviation for ductal carcinoma *in situ*.

DNA
Material found in the nucleus of all cells. Contains genetic information for cell division and cell growth.

donor site
Part of the body from which tissue is taken for transfer to another part of the body for reconstruction.

double blind
A research study in which neither the participants nor the researchers know which subjects are in the control group and which subjects are in the test group.

doubling time
The time required to double the number of cells in a group of cells or in a tumor. A short doubling time (under 100 days) indicates a fast-growing tumor.

dose-dense chemotherapy
A regimen that uses more frequent administration of chemotherapy.

drain
A plastic tube, usually attached to a bulb, placed into the surgical site to collect any draining blood or fluid for a few days following surgery.

ductal carcinoma in situ
A cancer inside breast ducts that has not grown through the wall of the duct into the surrounding tissues. Also known simply as DCIS.

edema
Excess fluid in a body part. Lymphedema is swelling of the arm as a result of scarring of the lymph ducts after radiation or surgery in the axilla.

estrogen
A female hormone secreted by the ovaries which is essential for menstruation, reproduction, and the development of secondary sex characteristics, such as breasts.

fibroadenoma
A noncancerous, solid tumor most commonly found in breasts of younger women.

fibroid
A tumor composed of fibers or fibrous tissues.

5-FU (5-fluorouracil)
A drug used to kill cancer cells. Also available in pill form under the name of Xeloda.

flap
A portion of tissue with its blood supply moved from one part of the body to another. Flaps of muscle, fat, and skin are frequently used to provide tissue for reconstructing breasts.

general anesthesia
Anesthesia which puts your whole body to sleep. Usually given through injection or gases.

genes
Areas on chromosomes that contain hereditary information that is transferred from cell to cell.

guided imagery
Using directed mental images to provide relaxation, mental healing, or higher levels of consciousness.

hemoglobin
A protein in blood which carries oxygen.

HER-2/neu
An oncogene which may help determine resistance to hormone and chemotherapy.

hormone
Chemical substance that helps regulate growth, metabolism, and reproduction.

immune system
System by which the body protects itself from outside invaders or internal defects.

immunotherapy
Therapy that works by enhancing the body's own defense system.

infiltrating ductal carcinoma
A cancer that began in a milk duct and has spread to areas outside the duct.

LCIS
Abbreviation for lobular carcinoma *in situ*.

linear accelerator
A machine that produces high energy X-ray beams to destroy cancer cells during radiation therapy.

lobular carcinoma in situ
A tumor confined to the milk-producing lobules of the breast (LCIS).

margin
The area of normal tissue surrounding a tumor when it is surgically removed.

metastatic cancer
Cancer which has spread beyond the breast to other parts of the body.

micro-surgery
Sewing together almost hair-thin blood vessels with the aid of a microscope.

mind-body connection
A philosophical theory that states that the mind can control bodily functions.

modified radical mastectomy
The most common type of mastectomy. Breast skin, nipple, areola, and some of the underarm lymph nodes are removed. The chest muscles are saved.

myo-cutaneous flap
A section of muscle, fat, and skin transferred for reconstruction of the breast

needle localization
A procedure in which a radiologist inserts a thin wire into the breast. Later, a surgeon will follow this wire to find the tumor.

Nolvadex (tamoxifen)
An anti-estrogen drug that may be given to women with estrogen receptor positive tumors.

non-surgical biopsy
A biopsy where samples of a lump or tumor are removed with a needle under local anesthesia.

oncogene
A gene that contributes to the malignant transformation of a cell.

oncologist
A physician who specializes in oncology—a specialty dealing with cancer treatment.

oral chemotherapy
Chemotherapy taken in pill form instead of by intravenous injection.

osteoporosis
Increased bone fragility that occurs with age, often due to lack of the female hormone estrogen.

PDQ
A source of information published by the National Cancer Institute which lists all clinical and experimental trials currently underway.

pectoralis muscles
Muscles located under the breast and attached to the front of the chest wall and extending to the upper arms.

port
A device surgically inserted under the skin of the chest, and connected to a very large vein, so that chemotherapy can be injected.

precancerous lesions
Abnormal cellular changes that are potentially capable of becoming cancer.

prednisone - (Deltasone, Orasone)
A steroid used to decrease inflammation; also used in combination with cytotoxic drugs.

progesterone
A female hormone produced by the ovaries during a specific time in the menstrual cycle that causes the breasts to prepare to produce milk.

prognosis
A prediction of the course of the disease; future prospect for the patient.

prosthesis
An artificial breast form worn inside a bra after a mastectomy.

protein
Complex compounds which hold amino acids essential for growth and repair of tissues.

radical mastectomy
Removal of entire breast, as well as underlying muscles, causing significant deformity. No longer performed today.

recurrence
Reappearance of cancer after a period of remission.

risk counselor
A trained healthcare professional who can advise a woman on her risk of developing breast cancer.

saline
A salt water solution,
1. given intravenously during surgery to maintain proper body functioning, or
2. used to fill a synthetic implant for breast reconstruction.

sentinel node
The single axillary lymph node that can be examined to determine if cancer has spread beyond the breast to other lymph nodes.

stem cell
Cells which will eventually become blood cell producers in the bone marrow.

stereotactic core needle biopsy
A biopsy performed using two mammographic views to pinpoint the site of the tumor.

suppressor gene
A gene that can reverse the effect of a specific type of mutation in other genes.

suture
A surgeon's stitch.

tamoxifen (Nolvadex)
An anti-estrogen drug that may be given to women with estrogen receptor positive tumors to block tumor cell growth.

taxanes
Taxol and Taxotere, drugs used for treatment of breast cancer

"tummy tuck"
A procedure in which a portion of fat and skin is removed from the abdomen, reducing the size of one's "tummy."

ultrasound
High frequency sound waves used to locate a tumor inside the body. Helps determine if a breast lump is solid or filled with fluid.

visualization
Forming a mental image of something not present to the sight. This technique can be used for relaxation or to help your body fight cancer.

Xeloda (5-FU)
A drug for treatment of advanced breast cancer. Xeloda is taken by mouth in pill form, rather than by intravenous injection.

QUESTIONS TO ASK YOUR HEALTHCARE PROVIDERS

The following are questions gathered from the book. They are broken down by chapters with space for your own notes. Feel free to tear or cut out these pages, and give them the person who will be accompanying you on your medical visits, to use as reminders of what you want to discuss.

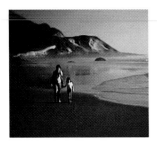

CHAPTER 1: FACING BREAST CANCER

What should I tell my loved ones about my condition?

Can you refer me to a counselor or to a support group specializing in breast cancer issues?

Could you give me the names of specialists you think I should see? How about another set of names so I can choose the specialist(s) I like best?

Is there a multidisciplinary breast cancer team in your facility?

Tell me about your experience in dealing with breast cancer.

Can you give me the name of a breast cancer expert who can give me a second opinion? Could you forward my chart, test results, and my biopsy slides to the doctor who is going to give me a second opinion?

Where can I find more information about breast cancer? Do you, or your clinic or hospital, have a resource center? A library?

CHAPTER 4: SURGERY

Questions to Ask Your Surgeon:

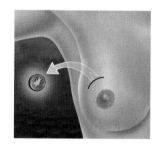

Is lumpectomy an option for me?   Why or why not?

Does a mastectomy decrease the chances of the cancer coming back?

How will my breast look after the treatment?   Can you show me pictures?

Can you refer me to a plastic surgeon so I can discuss my reconstruction options?

What kind of reconstruction procedure do you think would be best for me?

Who can I talk to about my concerns about appearance, dating, pregnancy, etc?

How much pain should I expect in the first few days after the procedure?

How long before I can go back to my regular activities?   Do I need to arrange to have someone help me with my daily activities?

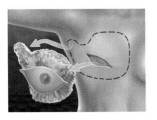

Do you recommend that I have a sentinel lymph node biopsy instead of a full axillary lymph node dissection? Why?

Are you and your surgical team experienced in performing this procedure?

Questions to Ask Your Anesthesiologist:

If I have general anesthesia, how long will it take me to get back to normal? What will I feel and hear if I have local anesthesia?

Will you give me something to control the pain after I wake up from the anesthetic?

CHAPTER 5: RECONSTRUCTION

Questions to Ask Your Plastic Surgeon:

What type of reconstruction do you think is best for me?

Will an implant make it more difficult to detect a local recurrence?

What should I know about the "skin-sparing" mastectomy?

What is the latest information regarding the safety of silicone implants?

Can you show me pictures of reconstruction procedures you have done?

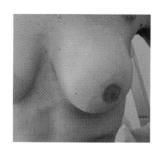

Could I meet with some of the women so I can see and feel their breasts?

Will my insurance pay for the reconstruction, even if it is done later? Will it pay for a breast prosthesis?

Will I have a lot of pain? How can the pain be treated?

Questions to Ask Your Insurance Company:

Does my policy cover the costs of the implant surgery, the implant anesthesia, and other related hospital costs? To what extent?

Does it cover treatments for medical problems that may be caused by the implant or the reconstruction?

Does it cover removal of the implants if this becomes necessary?

If I choose to delay reconstruction and my company changes insurance plans, will I still be covered for breast reconstruction at a later date?

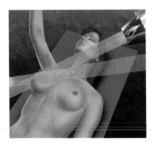

Chapter 6: Radiation Therapy

Why do I need radiation therapy?

How is the radiation oncologist (physician) involved if the treatments are given by the therapists?

How will I evaluate the effectiveness of the treatments?

Which method is better for me, external beam or brachytherapy?

Can I continue my usual work or exercise schedule?

Can I arrange to be treated elsewhere if I am traveling?

What side effects, if they occur, should I report immediately?

Can I expose the treated area to the sun?

Will I be able to conceive and bear a child after treatments?

What is the difference in cost between brachytherapy and external beam?

Chapter 7: Chemotherapy

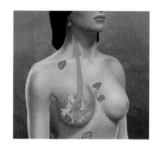

Do I need chemotherapy? Why?

What are the benefits and risks of chemotherapy? How successful is this treatment for the type of cancer I have?

How will you evaluate the effectiveness of the treatments?

What side effects will I experience?

Can I work while I'm having chemotherapy?

Can I travel between treatments (short business or pleasure trips)? What other limitations can I expect?

How can I manage nausea? Should I eat before I come for my treatments?

Will I continue to have my menstrual periods? If not, when will they return?

Should I use birth control? What type do you recommend?

Will I be able to conceive and bear a child after treatments?

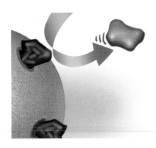

CHAPTER 8: HORMONE THERAPY

Did the tests on my tumor show that the cells were sensitive to hormones?
(Estrogen Receptor Positive, or Progesterone Receptor Positive)

Should I be treated with hormonal therapy or with chemotherapy, and why?

How will it affect my chance to have children?

How will it affect my sexual function?

What side effects should I expect?

Can I get pregnant while taking tamoxifen?

What birth control method would be most suitable to my lifestyle?

CHAPTER 9: IMMUNOTHERAPY

Is immunotherapy right for me?

Would I also benefit more from chemotherapy or hormonal therapy?

CHAPTER 10: COMPLEMENTARY AND ALTERNATIVE THERAPIES

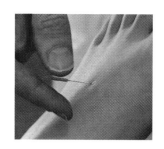

What benefits can be expected from this therapy?

What are the risks associated with this therapy? Do the known benefits outweigh the risks?

What side effects can be expected?

Will the therapy interfere with conventional treatment?

Will the therapy be covered by health insurance?

CHAPTER 11: DCIS

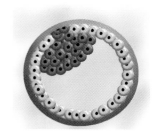

What grade is my DCIS?

How well will I do without radiation?

Do you work with a team that includes a mammographer and an experienced pathologist?

What is the downside of getting radiation after removal of the DCIS tumor?

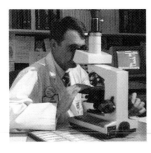

CHAPTER 12: CLINICAL TRIALS

How do I know the facility doing the study is reputable?

Are there other centers doing the same research on the same drugs or methods?

What is involved in terms of tests, treatments, and additional time commitments?

What results can be reasonably expected in my particular case?

What are the currently accepted treatments and how do they compare to the trial?

How can I be sure that I won't be under-treated, or miss the opportunity to be treated with established, conventional therapy?

What would my financial commitment be and how can I cope with it?

Will I need to be available for follow-up testing indefinitely?

Can I travel, work, or move to another city?

CHAPTER 13: LIFE AFTER CANCER

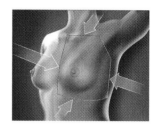

What can I do if I wake up at night worrying about my cancer?

Will the cancer cells that may have spread to other parts of my body start to grow when I stop taking chemotherapy?

Should my sisters get genetically tested?

Shouldn't we be doing more testing on me to make sure the cancer didn't come back?

What can I do about feeling excessively tired?

Why have I lost interest in intimate relations with my partner?

Why can't I sleep or relax or feel interested in anything?

Why can't I stop feeling that I am going to die because of the cancer?

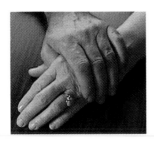

CHAPTER 14: A GUIDE FOR YOUR PARTNER

Do you have any pamphlets or videos about breast cancer we can take home and review?

Who would you recommend we see for a second opinion?

Can you put us in touch with women who you treated for breast cancer, and with their partners?

Will there be loss of sensation in the breast area?

Will chemotherapy cause her hair to fall out?

Can we see pictures of what the surgical scar could look like?

CHAPTER 15: ADVANCED BREAST CANCER

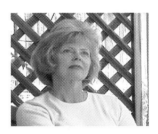

Where did my cancer spread?

If the tumor spread to other organs, is there any advantage to removing the tumor from the breast?

Do you recommend treatment with chemotherapy or radiation to shrink the tumor in the breast?

What tests need to be done on the tumor tissue to find the best treatment for it?

What clinical trials would be best suited to my case?

What support group should I join?

Index

MORE PRAISE FOR
Be a Survivor™

"This book does for the breast cancer survivor's mind what *Chicken Soup* does for the survivor's soul."

JACK CANFIELD, *Author*
Chicken Soup for the Surviving Soul

"Women and their partners will get a lot out of this CD-ROM. [It has] 12 hours of fact-packed information, given in scientific and lay terms."

JOURNAL OF THE
NATIONAL CANCER INSTITUTE

"Lives up to its title, and more. Geared toward breast cancer patients, their families and their support people, this CD-ROM could make all the difference in the attitude, and thus the recovery, of the patient facing breast cancer."

ADVANCE: FOR RADIOLOGIC
SCIENCE PROFESSIONALS

"A long-overdue book... 'One-stop shopping' for up-to-date, objective information that women need to make confident, informed decisions."

BETSY MULLEN, *survivor*
Founder, President, and CEO
WIN Against Breast Cancer

"A useful tool for patients and any lay person interested in breast cancer."

JOURNAL OF THE
AMERICAN MEDICAL ASSOCIATION

"An authoritative guide, illustrated with candid thoughts of breast cancer survivors."

WILLIAM H. GOODSON III, M.D.
Breast Surgeon

"A positive presentation of the essential facts every patient needs to know. Equally useful for the nurse and the family."

AMERICAN JOURNAL OF NURSING

"An excellent program that should help women face the difficult issues of cancer."

AMAN U. BUZDAR, M.D., *Author*
Ask the Doctor: Breast Cancer
M.D. Anderson Cancer Center

"The latest in the fight against breast cancer is as close as your home computer, and could save your life. It's realistic. It's informative. It's powerful. It's all on the new CD-ROM called "Be A Survivor.""

FOX NEWS

"For those ready to launch an all-out attack, *Be A Survivor* is a most empowering roadmap through the medical forest. It demystifies this disease. ...A loving guidebook through uncharted waters."

DOTTY EWING
Member of the Board,
WIN Against Breast Cancer